Medical Myths
Doctors Believe

Much of What Your Doctor Knows
is Untrue Or Unproven

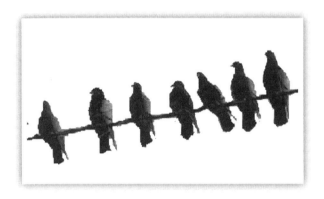

Like birds on a wire, most doctors get information from
each other or the drug companies,
not from reading real studies.

By

MICHAEL ANCHORS MD PHD

Copies are available from Amazon.com or from

Larryhobbs@cox.net or from . . .

Michael Anchors, M.D. Ph.D
16220 Frederick Rd., Suite 210
Gaithersburg MD 20877
Phone: 301-990-6061
Cell: 240-498-8380
Fax: 301-990-6064
E-mail: manchors@aol.com

ISBN: 146997486X

ISBN 13: 9781469974866

Table of Contents

Foreword

BY MALCOLM KENDRICK MD

Some time ago, I was looking through the latest definitions of various states of health. I can't remember why. I think I was writing a paper on multiple sclerosis and trying to establish the various stages that you may progress through, from fully fit and able to bed-bound and incapable of feeding yourself.

All types of health states were catalogued for all sorts of diseases. However, the really depressing definition was left to last. Someone with no disease or disability of any sort —— the type of person you or I might call "healthy" —— was defined as "temporarily able". As if health is a strange abnormal state, which, happily, given a bit of time, will revert to the more normal human condition of illness.

For some reason, this memory sprang into my mind when it was announced that the United Kingdom is going to introduce bowel-cancer screening for everyone between the ages of 60 and 70 as part of our new Brave New World of enforced healthiness for all. An announcement that left me profoundly depressed.

Despite my misgivings, however, I have to admit that, in general, most people seem ecstatic about the introduction of yet more health screening. It seems to be a self-evidently good thing. Pick up a disease early, especially cancer, and you can cure it. But if it were left for a few more years, it would be deadly. Who could possibly object to that? Anything that stops people from dying must be a good thing, mustn't it? Stop being an old curmudgeon.

I don't know....... Somehow all this screening and monitoring and treating things like raised blood pressure with drugs —— for the rest of your life —— seems to me to be in danger of stopping people from living, not dying. It may scem trite to say "no one gets out of life alive." This attitude is often dismissed as defeatist or nihilist. But I think it is critically important how our lives are lived —— not just how long they are.

Even from a purely practical perspective, I have doubts. If two million people are sent kits through the post to test for blood in the faeces (how lovely), around five percent will test positive. That is 100,000 positive tests. Around 90 percent of these will be false positive, by which I mean the test will come back positive for a variety of different reasons, not cancer.

So, 90,000 people will be scared witless. They will all undergo colonoscopy, an unpleasant and costly procedure, and then be pronounced "healthy" —— sort of. Despite this, many of them will become horribly worried and a certain number will suffer chronic anxiety. Believe me, I see them in my clinic every day.

If, on the other hand, you decide to throw the kit away in a fit of deranged personal liberty, you will be reminded and chided for years that you really should take the test —— it's for your own good, don't you know.

I don't know. There are always those who will say that even if one life is saved, it is worth any price. But I am not so sure. After all, we accept tens of thousands of deaths each year for the convenience of driving cars. Why won't we accept a few hundred more deaths a year for the freedom of living without added anxiety and fear in our lives?

If you screened everybody for every illness, everybody would be found to have an illness —— even if many of these findings would be false positive. And if everyone is ill, then everyone needs treatment of some sort. And I am not sure whether I want to live in a world where we are all considered to be ill, and under the command of the medical profession. For now, I am temporarily able and I would like to stay that way.

Acknowledgments

I could not have written this book without the help of Larry Hobbs, former editor of *Obesity Research Update* who maintains the blog at Fatnews.com. Larry reads widely and through his computers has access to, and gives the rest of us access to, the medical literature.

Only his modesty kept him from being a co-author on this book. The National Library of Medicine in Bethesda, Maryland, was good, too. I am fortunate to live near it.

My wife, attorney and all-around literate person, Laurel Anchors edited my drafts and clothed and fed me while I was afflicted with the writing disease. My daughter Rachel produced Figure 11 in this book, and daughter Lindsay produced the cover.

I acknowledge the wonderful existence of Joel Kauffman, Duane Graveline, Sid Port, Malcolm Kendrick, Nortin Hadler, Gary Taubes and many others, who, wandering in the limbo of official non-recognition, have continued to shout that the Emperor of Medicine has no clothes. The day will come when your contributions, gentlemen, will be recognized, and governments will fund real medical research turning scientists to useful work instead of being the toadies of the pharmaceutical companies. The companies, too, will benefit by selling real medicines that really work.

The main obstacle to progress is not ignorance, but the illusion of knowledge.

DANIEL BOORSTIN,
LIBRARIAN OF CONGRESS

❧

The besetting sin of America is wishful thinking.

ELEANOR ROOSEVELT

❧

True morality consists not in following the beaten track, but in finding out the true path for ourselves and fearlessly following it.

MOHANDAS GHANDI

CHAPTER 1

Most of what you know is wrong or at least there is no evidence for it, and you are being injured by the lack of true knowledge.

Most of what most people know, they know only because someone else told them so. And those people, in turn, knew only what someone else told them, and so on, back up the chain to what? to nothing usually.

Some of what you know you know from your own observations of life. Your observations may have been imperfect, some deductions off, but you still had a better chance of finding the truth doing your own thinking than by borrowing someone else's thinking.

Think For Yourself

It used to be the American way, but it is no more.

Fortunately most of the wrong things you know don't matter. For most of us, it doesn't matter whether the Earth is round or flat. You can sell insurance or bake a chocolate cake just as well believing the Sun is Apollo's chariot. But when it comes to your health, the wrong things you know matter a lot.

More than that, your doctor's ignorance hurts you. Most of what doctors know, they know only because the pharmaceutical companies told them so. Doctors themselvesare told not to trust their own observations, because those are said to be "anecdotal". Few doctors understand what anecdotal means, but they can tell by the tone of voice that it must be bad. Only big studies can define the truth, the pharmaceutical companies declare.

They *would* say that of course, since only they have the resources to fund large clinical trials. The U.S. government funds little research on its own. Nowadays most research projects at the NIH, where I used to work, are NIH/pharm company partnerships. The content of the big studies legally belongs to the pharmaceutical companies. They can publish it, alter it or suppress it at will. What do you suppose they do?

In a way it's moot since few physicians read clinical studies anyway. Few know how. The skill is not taught in medical school. I was trained as both an M.D. and a Ph.D. I have seen both patterns of education. Physicians are taught a list of facts; PhDs are taught how to think. I swear, the *Journal of the American Medical Association* arrives in every U.S. physician's mailbox and thirty minutes later, it's in the trash. Doctors, especially primary doctors, get their information from the people who give them notepads and stethoscopes. American doctors are not paid to study; they are paid to work.

Europe has changed its ways. The Netherlands developed the first mandatory system of continuing medical education and retesting. Germany developed a good system that has been the model for many countries.[1] France replaced their old failed voluntary system with a new mandatory system in 2009.[2]

But America has continued its policy of not retesting doctors. Primary care doctors widely bypass the voluntary system of CME (continuing medical education) credits. Some surgical and medical specialty boards require retesting, but–you will laugh at this–most of the CME materials are prepared by the pharmaceutical companies. The circle is closed.

The American medical journals are no longer supported by subscription fees. Doctors no longer subscribe to journals, and the medical libraries outside of universities or Washington DC have vanished. True, you can get the abstracts of clinical studies on the Internet, but the abstracts present a rosy view of the results and omit important details.

The journals are now supported almost entirely by advertising placed by pharmaceutical companies. The journals are filled with pretty pictures, as in *Glamour* and *Vogue*. But there is no way a journal will publish any article critical of their sponsors or their products. For a while, *Archives of Internal Medicine* held out, publishing letters from skeptics[3]; but when the editor retired, they too switched to the majority policy. What does freedom of speech mean in a country where money controls the public megaphone?

It doesn't have to be this way. Your doctor, and YOU, could read excellent books on your own, books such as Joel Kauffman's *Malignant Medical Myths* (Infinity Publishing, 2006) exposing the dangerous mistakes that cost so many lives and so much treasure. Joel's book is not the only good work–there are others.

Most of you would find Kauffman's book tough sledding. I did. Joel is a PhD chemist and statistician. You need some introduction to his methods before launching in. This book is the introduction you need. It may be the only book you need. In this book I have dealt with much of Joel's material. I disagreed with him on a few points, and I have added some new ideas. Joel's book dates from 2006. This book is from 2011.

In this book the discussion of each medical myth is handled in a six-part format.

The Myth
The Fact
Why we should have known better

How we got confused
What to do now
References

Before we get to the myths, I must teach you the meaning of scientific *evidence*, because everything we truly know is based on evidence. Let's begin with what scientific evidence is *not*.

- Scientific evidence is not the pronouncements of experts. Nothing is true only because someone said so, or because everyone said so. Evidence is not the beliefs of an Age.
- Evidence is not the age of a belief either. Precedent plays no role in science.
- Evidence is not the reasonableness of a belief or the power of faith.
- Evidence is not the absence of counter-evidence. Nothing is true by default.

Instead, scientific evidence is only two things.

- Well-done scientific experiments
- Extensive long-term practical experience accurately observed by many people (also called empirical knowledge)

I have more to say about this, but I suspect you are eager to get to the myths. So let's head out! Let's tackle two simple questions first.

1. For all the effort to control blood pressure, cholesterol and blood sugar, have we reduced the number of heart attacks?
2. For all the cancer research, are we curing cancer more often?

References

1. Pozniak E Silber D. The state of CME in Europe. PharmaNews 2008;7(8):1-3.
2. http://www.legifrance.gouv.fr/ Sorry it's in French. I can't find a translation.
3. The word "skeptic" comes from the Greek verb 'skep-tomai', meaning to think. Skepticism, therefore, is good.

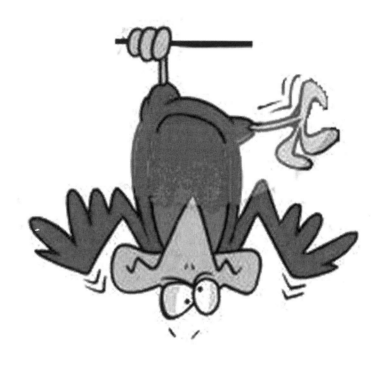

The Myths

MYTH #1

Heavy emphasis on preventive medicine in recent decades has reduced the number of Americans who have a heart attack each year.

Fact

Not.

Why We Should Have Known Better

Because heart attack is still the leading cause of death in late middle-age men and women in the U.S., despite all the diet advice and statin drugs doctors have given.[1] You expect very old people to die from something of course, but what's up with so many middle-aged people still dying from heart attack?

Since heart attack was so far ahead in first place, we might have had some improvement in mortality, i.e death rate, without knocking heart attack out of the #1 spot; but in fact, the annual incidence of heart attacks in U.S. *non-smokers* has scarcely declined. What improvements we have seen in mortality have come from people quitting smoking.[2] What we got for so much attention to blood pressure and cholesterol was bupkis.

How We Got Confused

Because to this day we still don't know the true cause of heart attacks. Sure the most common scenario is a fresh blood clot blocking a coronary blood vessel, i.e. a vessel on the surface of the heart, interrupting the flow of blood and oxygen to the heart, but what leads to that? Why are the atherosclerotic plaques only at arterial branch-points? Why don't veins get atherosclerosis?[3] We know so little because all the scientists and funding piled into the cholesterol boat. We backed too many "experts" and not enough skeptics.

We have reduced the death rate from heart attacks in the hospital setting by more accurate detection, the use of blood thinners and better control of arrhythmias; but *the actual number* of heart attacks per 100,000 people has stayed about the same.[4,5,6,7] That is not an easy statement to make, so I included a lot of references.

There are some reasons why heart attacks in late-middle-age people would have gone up. (1) Better detection of heart attacks in women and minorities. (2) The rise in obesity and diabetes. (3) The decline in personal income for all but the most wealthy Americans and the resulting stress for everyone else.[8,9]

There was even a big reason for heart attacks to go down–the decline in smoking.[10] Smoking rates dropped from 43% in 1970 to 22% in 2007.

Looking on the bright side you might think that if low-fat diet and controlling blood pressure and cholesterol did not reduce the overall rate of heart attacks *in non-smokers*, maybe the situation would have been worse without them. We might have had more heart attacks. Hmm. Maybe.

But is that the best you can say for the statin drugs which cost us $18 billion dollars annually? And all the blood pressure pills and the fat-free food? The best you can say is, maybe it would have been worse without them? I wanted more than that from medicine and science after so much money and time spent.

What To Do Now?

The easy pickings in Medicine have been picked. Antibiotics. Vaccines. Soap. Any further progress against the diseases that attack Americans will require us to stop wasting money on colonial wars and space exploration and focus instead on biomedical research. The allocation of money to science cannot be linked to politics or to corporate welfare for pharmaceutical companies.[11,12]

We need to do a better job of teaching scientific method to our scientists We must reward studies with a negative result as generously as those with a positive result. The truth itself is never either positive nor negative–it is only just what it is. The proper goal of science is to find the truth. We must put money into science without having our scientists controlled by money.

References

I am not going to burden this book with too many references. I give only enough references for readers to know that I'm not making stuff up and I actually read the references. At least one reference for each myth has an extensive bibliography. I give many Internet sites so you can look things up quickly. It is a sign of the times that few doctors even have access to a medical library.

1. http://www.cdc.gov/NCHS/data/nvsr/nvsr58/nvsr58_19.pdf
2. http://www.cdc.gov/mmwr/preview/mmwrhtml/mm5751a1.htm
3. *The Great Cholesterol Con* by Malcolm Kendrick, John Blake Publishing, London, 2007
4. Goldberg RJ, Yarzebski J, Lessard D et al. A two-decades (1975 to 1995) long experience in the incidence, in-hospital and long-term case-fatality rates of acute myocardial infarction: a community-wide perspective. *J Am Coll Cardiol.* 1999; 33: 1533-1539.
5. Sytkowski PA D'Agostino RB Belanger et al. Secular Trends in Long-term Sustained Hypertension, Long-term Treatment, and Cardiovascular Mortality. The Framingham Heart Study 1950 to 1990. *Circulation* 1996;93:697-703.
6. Parikh NI Gona P Larson MG et al. Long-Term Trends in Myocardial Infarction Incidence and Case Fatality in the National Heart, Lung, and Blood Institute's Framingham Heart Study. *Circulation.* 2009;119:1203-1210.

7. Yeh RW Go AS. Rethinking the Epidemiology of Acute Myocardial Infarction. Challenges and Opportunities. *Arch Intern Med.* 2010;170:759-764.
8. Reich R. *Aftershock* Vintage Press, New York, 2010
9. Pierson P Hacker JS. *Winner Take All Politics* Simon & Schuster, New York, 2010.
10. http://www.cdc.gov/mmwr/preview/mmwrhtml/ mm5751a1.htm
11. Petersen M. *Our Daily Medicines.* Sarah Crichton Book, New York, 2008.
12. Angell M. *The Truth About The Drug Companies.* Random House, New York, 2004.

MYTH #2

Heavy emphasis on cancer research has led to more effective treatments. Overall, 60% of cases of cancer are cured by treatment now.

Fact

Bullfeathers.

Why We Should Have Known Better

The anti-cancer treatments used in practice now are still surgery, ionizing radiation, and chemotherapy, the same treatments we have had since 1965. The more promising immunologic treatments, targeting cancer cells and sparing normal cells, are not yet available.

How We Got Confused

By being vague about the definition of a "cure". Any layperson assumes the word means the cancer is gone; it will never kill the patient or cause disfigurement and pain again. But when doctors and medical researchers think about cure, they think in terms of the five-year survival rate. If the patient is still alive five years after the treatment, they consider the patient cured. The reason they think this way is because the five-year survival rate is the only published data they have to go on.

But you would not consider that your aunt who died from breast cancer six years after her treatment was cured, would you? Or that your dad was cured of prostate cancer by getting radioactive pellets in his prostate. He continued to suffer from bone fractures for years afterward, and from radiation damage to his bladder. That's a strange kind of cure.

It is true that the five-year survival for many cancers has increased.

TABLE 1.

CHANGES IN 5-YEAR SURVIVAL RATES FOR 20 TYPES OF SOLID TUMORS. DATA FROM WELCH ET AL. (I HAVE SELECTED FOUR, TO COMPARE WITH TABLE 2)

	1950-54	**1989-95**
Breast	60%	86%
Prostate	43	93
Lung	6	14
Colon	41	62

But the main reason for this apparent improvement is that we have been finding cancers earlier in their course. The patient still dies at the same stage of the disease on the same fated day of the calendar. We haven't delayed the final stage of the disease or averted death when it was destined to occur. We only improved the five-year survival rate by having more people die at 7 and 8 years after the initial diagnosis instead of at 4 or 5 years. That is a triumph of detection, not a triumph of treatment.

TABLE 2.

TEN-YEAR SURVIVAL RATES FOR PATIENTS ON CHEMOTHERAPY FOR COMMON METASTATIC CANCERS. FROM BLECH ET AL.

Time Period	Original cancer location of Treatment			
	Breast	Prostate	Lung	Colon
1978-1986	11%	—	3%	4%
1987-1993	8	2	1	5
1994-2002	7	3	2	5

As for prevention. Well. Reducing smoking certainly reduced lung cancer. Good! But mammograms have not been effective (see Myth #17). And sun screens have not reduced the incidence of melanoma. The same number of people get melanoma as before, because they are genetically programmed to get it. Sun screens succeed only in blocking the production of cancer-protective vitamin D in the skin. A little sun is good for you. Only the people who listen to doctors get confused. Try avoiding the sun completely and you'll see–you will get depressed and sick.

It is not enough for doctors to give medical advice on the basis of what they reasonably expect from theory or guessing. They are paid to be real experts–they *should be* real experts. And the only way to become a real expert is by reading scientific evidence. No doctor should ever say anything to a patient beyond "good morning" except on the basis of scientific evidence.

What To Do Now?

Accelerate the work on immunologic treatments of cancer, i.e. using the body's immune system to kill or contain cancer. Stop wasting money on chemotherapy, radiation treatments or mammograms. With all the time and money we spent on those things, if they were going to work, they would have.

Stop hyping results. The cure rate for cancer is not 60%.

The funding of research should not be linked to success, because then scientists are forced to claim success in any way possible to keep their funding. They know it is possible to publish *and* perish. You can perish by publishing negative results, even though, as I said, negative results are as important as positive ones. Any honest result should be rewarded. No phony or over-hyped result ever should be.

References

1. Kauffman J. *Malignant Medical Myths*. Infinity Publishing, 2006, pages 219-258.
2. Welch HG. *Should I Be Tested For Cancer? Maybe Not and Here's Why*. University of California Press, Berkeley CA, 2004
3. Blech J. Giftkur Ohne Nützen. *Der Spiegel* 2004;4(41):160-162.

CHAPTER 2
More About Evidence

Back in Chapter 1, I was explaining scientific evidence when I got worried that technical explanations might be boring and unnecessary. After all, if doctors already did a good job of curing heart disease and cancer, you wouldn't need to know about randomized trials and p values. If plumbers did a good job of fixing toilets (they do), you wouldn't need to know about toilets. You don't need to learn to knit if you can buy sweaters at the store. That is what civilization means–each of us specializes in producing a product or service for other people, relying on others to provide the products and services we need. You trusted doctors to provide medical services and pharmaceutical companies to produce medicines. How has that worked out for you? We asked two simple questions . . .

1. For all the effort to control blood pressure, cholesterol and blood sugar have we reduced the number of heart attacks?
2. For all the cancer research are we curing cancer more often?

It turned out that the risk of heart attacks has not decreased since smoking declined, and the improved cure rate of cancer, in general, was a mirage (with some exceptions).

So it seems we need to read scientific papers for ourselves since the doctors don't read, and decide for ourselves what treatments work. Perhaps if we did that, we would shame the physicians into doing more reading themselves.

If you find it hard to believe that American doctors don't read the scientific literature, please go to www.PubMed and search for "J Avorn". Avorn and his colleagues at the Harvard School of Public Health have published a twenty year series of articles exploring the disconnect between scientific knowledge and physician practice.

To do any reading for yourself, you will need to learn some scientific methods and statistics. I will teach you a little in this chapter, and I promise, it won't be hard. After that lesson, we'll get back to the myths.

Scientific experiments as evidence

The best experiments in medicine are large, long, randomized double-blind placebo-controlled trials (DBP) done by qualified people with no financial interest in the outcome of the study. Such studies are rare. Usually, we must settle for a standard of evidence short of the gold standard DBP.

Just so you know . . .

- "large", in the above, means thousands of subjects in the study. The more important the topic, the larger the study should be.
- "long" means long enough to get a statistical significant result
- "randomized" means the study subjects were randomly assigned to receive the treatment or the placebo.
- "double-blind" means that neither the doctors nor the subjects knew whether they received the real treatment or the placebo.

- "placebo-controlled". The patients in the control group received an inactive substitute indistinguishable from the real thing.

DBPs are a specific example of a *prospective* study. The other type of study in the world is a *retrospective* study. Prospective studies are better than retrospective studies.

In a **prospective study** a group of subjects is given a treatment first and the results are measured later.

In a **retrospective study** the treatment had already been used by the subjects before the study ever commenced.

All DBP studies are, by definition, prospective, but not all prospective studies are DBPs. The study by Stolarz et al. in Myth #3 was a prospective study that is not a DBP. In that study a random selection of adults was followed for 9 years. During that time their sodium excretion was measured, and the number of heart attacks and cases of high blood pressure recorded. Urinary sodium excretion was used as a marker for how much sodium was in their diet. The study found that salt in the diet did not raise blood pressure or cause heart attacks. That was a prospective study, but not a DBP study.

The more general term for this best class of studies, the prospective studies, is a **randomized controlled trial** (RCT). The Stolarz study was an RCT. Randomized control trials are better than retrospective studies.

Now let's talk about the different types of retrospective studies.

In a **case-control study,** a small group of patients with a disease is paired with a control group of people without the disease. Both groups are asked if they previously received any of a list of treatments, or followed any of a list of habits. If the group with the disease more often had a listed treatment, or habit, than the control group did, the study suggests that the treatment or habit was associated with the disease.

It could work the other way. If the treatment or habit was more common in the *control* group than in the disease group, you would think the treatment or habit was not associated with the disease.

Case-control studies are commonly used to study rare diseases, for which it is impractical to assemble enough patients to do a prospective study. Case-control studies are cheap, and easy.

An example of a case-control study is the study showing that patients in the hospital after a heart attack are more likely to have brushed their teeth twice a day than control patients. (BMJ 2010; 340:c2451) Can you conclude that frequent tooth-brushing prevents heart attacks? Not at all. You will see why in a moment.

A second type of retrospective study is the **epidemiological study**. In these studies the prevalence of a disease in a population, usually a gender, race or nation, is noted–call that, fact A. Then the presence of some other factor such as diet or climate or habits is noted–call that, fact B. If we see that where B is high, A is high also, and where B is low, A is low, then we say there is a correlation between B and A. An inverse correlation is also possible; A could be high where B is low, etc.

An example. In some countries where people eat a high-fat diet, heart attacks are common. In other countries where people eat less fat, heart attacks are less common. We can say that in those countries, there is a correlation between fat intake and heart attacks.

Unfortunately many people think such a study shows that eating fat *causes* heart attacks, and that is not correct. Please, please, learn the following . . .

Retrospective studies can never prove causation.

Only prospective studies furnish evidence for causation.
So many people do not understand this. Let's say that in a retrospective study, when A was true, B was also true.

You cannot say from that fact that A *caused* B, because both A and B might have both been the result of a third element C. For instance, if people eating more fat were more likely to smoke (fact C), then you would have seen the same result, i.e fat-eaters getting more heart attacks, even though it was the smoking that caused the heart attacks and not the fat. The retrospective study design did not identify the true cause. And there could have been a factor D and an E, and an F in the mix, too. You don't know. It really is hopeless.

The prospective study design, on the other hand, gets rid of the mess. In the prospective study, the experimental group and the control group are matched for everything except the single parameter being studied. The C's and D's and E's all cancel out.

* * *

A final group of retrospective studies to mention is the **meta-analysis**, a study of studies. The author collects and compares a large number of different studies on a single topic. There are many meta-analyses in the literature, and we need them; but they are only as good as the studies the authors review, and only good if they collect most of the good studies. The most common failing of meta-analyses is **selection bias**; the authors include more studies favoring their favorite point of view and omit studies with results opposed to their ideas. Watch out for selection bias.

* * *

The **prevalence** of a disease is the number of people in a population at any time who have had the disease of interest *at some time* now or in the past. The prevalence is an effort to estimate the amount of the factor in the population causing a particular disease, whether it be germs, toxins or whatever else.

The **incidence** is the number of people in the population developing the active disease in a specific time period, usually a year. The incidence is a measure of the burden of the disease on people and on the health care system.

People get these two terms mixed up. Often it doesn't matter, but sometimes it does.

* * *

One of my pet peeves is that Americans use the word "theory" as if it meant "guess". But a **guess** is just a guess, and only that. After experiments have shown support for a guess, the guess may become a **hypothesis**. Years later after many experiments and experience have supported the hypothesis and no crippling counter-evidence has surfaced, the hypothesis matures into a **theory**. But even then, a theory is not the truth. The truth is an unreachable goal, like the perfect martini. A theory is the closest human beings get to the real truth, outside of mathematics.

So in the future don't say you have a theory about where you left your sunglasses. Say, you can guess where they are.

* * *

Moving on. The **p value** is the result of a statistical test on the data comparing one group to another. There are many such tests and the relevant value is not always called "p", but in general, if the p value equals 0.01, there is a one-in-a-hundred chance that the observed difference between the two groups occurred from random chance rather than from any real difference between the groups. P values are often written with a " < ". P<0.01 means there is better than a 99/100 chance that the observed difference was real.

Generally speaking, only p values of 0.01 or less are considered *statistically significant*. It should be so. We use these tests to make decisions about giving medicines to hundreds of thousands of people. We should not stake people's life on a p value of 0.02 or one in fifty. You think I'm kidding? If a study promises big profits for the pharmaceutical companies, they consider even p=.05 significant! There's an example in Myth #3.

* * *

The news that retrospective studies, i.e. most published studies, cannot establish causality was the first big news of this chapter. Here is the second big news . . .

Relative risk is meaningless without knowing the absolute risk.

To calculate the relative risk reduction, for heart attack–to take an example–you compare the total number of heart attacks in the drug-treated group with the number in the placebo group, *no matter how many people were in the two groups.* In a hypothetical study of 2000 patients, it might happen that 11 people in the placebo group suffered a heart attack compared to 8 in the group receiving a statin drug. The relative risk reduction was thus 11 minus 8 divided by 11 = 27%. That sounds good, doesn't it?

The absolute rate of heart attacks in the placebo group was 11 divided by 1000 = 0.11%. That means 99.89% of the placebo subjects did not get a heart attack during the study. The relative rate of heart attacks in the statin group was 0.08%. In that group 99.99% did not get a heart attack. So you see, the statin drug reduced the actual incidence of heart attack by only 0.1%, probably not significant and certainly not worth the expense, risk and side-effects of statin drugs.

If relative risk really mattered, cyanide would be the best drug to prevent heart attack! In the placebo group 11 of 1000 patients would have a heart attack; in the cyanide group, NONE of the patients would have had a heart attack, because they all died from cyanide first. That's a relative risk reduction of heart attack of 100%. But the absolute risk reduction of death would be zero. Clearly absolute risk reduction is the crucial comparison, not relative risk.

But drug company representatives use relative risk reduction, instead of absolute risk reduction, to confuse doctors and clench the sale.

Take a real example, the WOSCOPS i.e. West of Scotland Trial, the main trial on which doctors rely to prescribe statin drugs to reduce cholesterol. At the end of that five-year trial 95.9% of the placebo patients were still alive, versus 96.8% of the patients who had taken the statin drug. The *absolute risk reduction* with the statin drug after five years was thus 96.8% - 95.9% = 0.9%. Paltry.

The *relative risk reduction* was . .
Data:
statin group: 100 - 96.8 = 3.2% died
placebo group: 100 - 95.9 = 4.1% died

Relative risk reduction = (4.1 - 3.2)/4.1 = .22 or 22%

It may be more clear with a 2 x 2 box . . .

	lived	**died**
statin	A 96.8%	B 3.2%
placebo	C 95.9%	D 4.1%

Then
absolute risk reduction = A - C = 96.8% - 95.9% = 0.9%

$$\text{relative risk reduction} = \frac{D - B}{D} = \frac{4.1\% - 3.2\%}{4.1\%} = 22\%$$

The drug rep says the risk reduction with the statin drug was 22%, because it sounds better than saying 0.9%. But is that honest? After five years of the study, 95.9% of the placebo patients were still alive and they were $2520 richer because they had not spent $1.40 a pill for pravastatin. 96.8% of the statin patients were still alive, too; but only 0.9% of them could attribute their survival to pravastatin.

The *absolute risk reduction* was the number you needed to know.

Sorry to spend so much time on this subject, but you need to understand it. Substituting *relative risk reduction* for *absolute risk reduction* is the most common error in determining a trial's significance.

* * *

There is a concept called *number needed to treat* (NNT). It is the inverse of the absolute risk reduction. For instance if a medicine provides an absolute reduction of death = 0.1%, then the number of people needed to treat to save one life is the inverse of 0.1 = 1000. I won't make a big deal about the NNT because Americans are not used to thinking this way. They will spend any amount of money to save one life (of the right type of people) or one treasured pet or one foreign country with oil. Their decisions are not based on budgeting.

* * *

Now I must make a confession. I played a trick on you a page back, a trick often used by the drug reps. Without telling you, I switched from discussing reduction in the risk of dying from a heart attack (the first hypothetical example) to the risk of dying from *any cause* (in the WOSCOPS trial discussion). If you didn't notice the switch, don't feel bad–most people don't notice.

The statin drugs do, indeed, reduce heart attacks a little, but they *increase* deaths from other causes, as I will show in Myth #5. The two effects cancel out. As a patient looking at a drug study, you don't really care if a drug reduces the chance of dying from heart attack if it doesn't reduce the chance of dying overall. If all a drug does is to switch the manner of death, what good is it? After all, heart attack is not a bad way to go; I'd rather die from that, than from cancer. In statin trials the cancer rate goes up.

So finally, here are the things you want to know from the drug reps . . .

- What is the absolute reduction of the risk of death from any cause?
- What is the statistical significance of the reduction, i.e. what was the p value?
- What are the side effects? What is the cost?

You will have a hard time getting that information from them, though they will be happy to furnish you with pens, stethoscopes and show tickets.

MYTH #3

A high-salt diet causes high blood pressure and heart attacks.

Fact

High-salt diet does not cause high blood pressure or hypertension (same thing). A low-salt diet actually increases heart attack deaths.

Why we should have known better

For thousands of years human beings salted food to preserve it.[1] Roman soldiers on the march were paid in salt; that's

24

why your pay is called "salary". Until recently human beings in most places ate a high sodium diet, but the rate of heart attacks was low. High blood pressure and heart attacks didn't take off until the advent of smoking, obesity, caffeine and too much sugar. Nicotine is an arterial constrictor and caffeine a cardiac stimulant. The fructose in sucrose and high-fructose corn syrup is a vasoconstrictor. Fructose increases the production of uric acid reducing nitric oxide production. Nitric oxide is a vasodilator.[2,3] Obesity increases blood pressure through many mechanisms.[4] You don't need to blame sodium; we have enough other reasons for high blood pressure.

How we got confused

By relying on epidemiological studies, which cannot show causation, and doing only limited prospective studies.[5] And by being content to guess about the mechanism of high blood pressure. Doctors assumed that since sodium increases blood pressure in patients with impaired kidney function, who can't excrete sodium, sodium might increase blood pressure in people with normal kidneys as well. Indeed when diuretics were given to people with functioning kidneys to increase the excretion of sodium, blood pressure did, indeed, go down, some, at first, in most people, though it usually returned to its former level in a few weeks.

When small prospective studies were done, they showed a variable response of blood pressure to sodium in the short term (weeks).[6,7,8] Some people, especially those with metabolic syndrome, i.e. central obesity and diabetes, seemed to have salt-sensitive blood pressure.[9] But no one followed the patients long enough to see if the blood pressure stayed elevated.

In most people, sodium did not raise the blood pressure even in the short-term. Critics said the studies weren't long enough. Okay. Then why not do longer studies?

In fact, a definitive *prospective* study was not published until March 2011, and it was done by European researchers not funded by a pharmaceutical company.[10] Stolarz et al.

showed that high-sodium diet did *not* lead to hypertension at all, and people taking in *less* sodium suffered *more* heart attack deaths, not fewer.

The study published in the March 4, 2011, edition of *Journal of American Medical Association* involved 3681 study participants followed for a mean duration of 8 years. The patients, randomly selected, were a cross-section of the western European adult population. They were not told what to eat; they ate what they wanted. The researchers measured the subjects' 24 hour urinary sodium excretion at intervals and measured their blood pressure.

Measuring the amount of sodium excreted in the urine in 24 hours is the best way to measure daily sodium intake because the body in equilibrium excretes all the sodium it takes in. There's no other good way to do the study. You can't ask people how much sodium they eat–they don't know. And it would have been hard for the researchers to tally everything the subjects ate and drank.

In the Katarzyna study, in the lowest third of sodium intake there were 50 deaths (4.1% of the group), in the middle third there were 24 deaths (1.9%) and in the highest third there were 10 deaths (0.8%) over the 8 year period. The *absolute reduction of risk of death* was 4.1 - 0.8 = 3.3%, and the p value was <.001 !

Recall that in the best statin study, there was an *absolute risk reduction* of only 0.9% with p value <.05. The WOSCOPS trial was a 4 year study and the Katarzyna trial 8 years, so you have to double the statin *absolute risk reduction* to compare it to the sodium *absolute risk reduction*. But the sodium *absolute risk reduction* 3.3% still beats the statin 1.8%. If sodium was a drug, you would use it, instead of a statin, to prevent death! It's twice as effective and costs less.

The abstract from the Katarzyna study says . . .

"In this population-based cohort, systolic blood pressure, but not diastolic pressure changes over time aligned with changes in sodium excretion, but this association did not translate into a higher risk of hypertension or CVD (cardiovascular disease). *Lower sodium excretion was associated with higher CVD mortality.* [italics added]"

The "association" in this study counts as evidence of actual causation, i.e. evidence hat low sodium *caused* more CVD deaths, because Katarzyna et al. was a prospective study.

By the way, the average daily sodium intake in the European study was 4.5 grams for men and 3.6 grams for women, about the same as for Americans (2.9–4.2 grams).[6]

You should look at that reference #11 from the CDC. What a load of cookies! It starts off . . .

"Excessive dietary sodium consumption increases blood pressure, **[oh yeah? based on what?]** which increases the risk for stroke, coronary heart disease, heart failure, and renal disease.**[?]** Based on *predictive modeling* of the health benefits of reduced salt intake on blood pressure, a population-wide reduction in sodium of 1,200 mg/day would reduce the annual number of new cases of coronary heart disease, etc."

Don't believe anything in medicine based on "predictive modeling". On climate-change perhaps. Geology maybe But in medicine, only randomized controlled trials count.

America could have done a good study like the Katarzyna study, twenty years sooner, but didn't. Why not? Look at all the hokum on sodium and blood pressure we did produce. America could have done the study first, but we were too focused on making pills and profits for Big Pharma.

What to do now?
Stop telling people to reduce the salt in their diet below the level they find palatable, and resolve to never again tell people to change their behavior without an adequate prospective study to back up the recommendation. If the U.S. economy keeps deteriorating, we will be paying our workers in salt anyway, their *salarium*, as the Romans did. Let them eat some of it.

References

1. *Salt* by Mark Kurlansky. Penguin Press, NY, 2003.
2. *Good Calories, Bad Calories* by Gary Taubes. Alfred Knopf, NY, 2007.
3. Lustig R. Sugar: The Bitter Truth. http://www.youtube.com/watch?v=dBnniua6-oM
4. Kurukulasuriya LR Stas S Lastra G et al. Hypertension in Obesity. *Endocrinol Metab Clin North Am* 2008; 37(3):647-62.
5. Intersalt Cooperative Research Group. Intersalt: an international study of electrolyte excretion and slood pressure. Results of 24 hour urinary sodium and potassium excretion. *BMJ* 1988;297:319-328.
6. Stamler EP Nichols J et al. Intersalt Cooperative Research Group. Intersalt revisited: further analyses of 24 hour sodium excretion and blood pressure with and across populations. *BMJ* 1996;312:1249-1253.
7. Sacks FM Svetkey LP Vollmer WM et al; DASH Sodium Collaborative Research Group. Effects of reduced dietary sodium and the Dietary Approaches to Stop Hypertension (DASH) diet. *NEJM* 2001;344:3-10.
8. Alderman MH. Dietary Sodium and Cardiovascular Health in Hypertensive Patients: The Case against Universal Sodium Restriction. *J Am Soc Nephrol* 2004:15;S47-S50.
9. Chen J Gu D Huang J Rao DC Jaquish CE Hixson JE Chen C-S Chen J Lu F Hu D, Rice T, N'Kelly T, Hamm L Whelton PK He J Metabolic syndrome and salt sensitivity of blood pressure in non-diabetic people in China: a dietary intervention study. *Lancet* 2009;373:829-835.
10. Stolarz-Skrzypek K, Kuznetsova T, Lutgarde T et al. Fatal and nonfatal outcomes, incidence of hypertension and blood pressure changes in relation to urinary sodium excretion. *JAMA* 2011;305:1777-1789.
11. CDC website http://www.cdc.gov/mmwr/preview/ mmwrhtml/ mm5924a4.htm

MYTH #4

High blood pressure causes heart attacks, and lowering blood pressure prevents them.

Fact

Sorry. No. Not in general. But it might help people in the top 10% for blood pressure. We don't really know.

Why we should have known better

Despite all the blood pressure reduction we have achieved, heart attacks are still the leading cause of death in the U.S.

The systolic blood pressure in healthy people who never get a heart attack increases normally with age; the old rule of thumb was BP = the age + 100. The idea of treating everyone, regardless of age, with a BP > 140/90 is saying that more than half the adult population over 40 has a disease called hypertension. More than half! Can that be right? We are medicalizing the nation. No one is normal! Everyone is to be taking a medicine. Won't that make the pharm companies happy?

You can't call being normal a disease.

Moreover women, as they age, have higher blood pressure than men, yet they have fewer heart attacks. Explain that!

How we got confused

By using the wrong statistical model to fit the Framingham data. The scientists drew a line that did not match the points on the graph and came to the wrong conclusions. Sid Port alerted us to this problem.[1]

The Framingham Study was our wonderful study of the entire population of Framingham, Massachusetts over a forty-year period cataloguing almost every measurable variable of life, data which we have mishandled in the case of hypertension (this myth) and cholesterol (the myth coming next).

Here is the data from the Framingham Study comparing deaths to blood pressure.

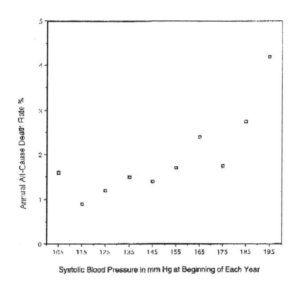

FIGURE 1.

MORTALITY VERSUS SYSTOLIC BLOOD PRESSURE. FRAMINGHAM STUDY

Looking at the graph, you think first that it shows that the higher the blood pressure, the more the deaths. You see what you expect to see. But take away the dot at SBP=195. Does the rest of the data look like a rising curve?

If the data did show a rising curve, you would be tempted to think that high blood pressure *causes* heart attacks, but you must not think that way. I taught you that retrospective studies never prove causality. And the graph doesn't say what the people died from. They might have died from heart attack, strokes, cancer or falling through the floor.

The points jump around a lot, too, don't they? Scientists are accustomed to drawing a smooth curve that comes close to most of the dots. This is the line the Framingham scientists drew.

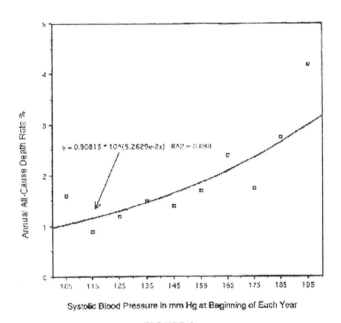

FIGURE 2.
THE SAME FRAMINGHAM DATA FITTED WITH A SMOOTH CURVE
BY LINEAR REGRESSION

I'm not kidding. This is the graph from which doctors came up with the recommendation to treat everyone regardless of age with a BP over 140/90. But do you think the line is a good fit to the data? Doesn't it bother you that some important points, such as the one at 195, fall so far off the line? In fact, it's a terrible fit! The R value is only 0.7. The R value is a measure of the quality of the fit.

Mother Nature doesn't care about smoothness of lines. She is unembarrassed about being complex. To properly fit the data you have to use two mathematical curves. Sid Port did the Framingham calculations again, properly, and this is what he saw.

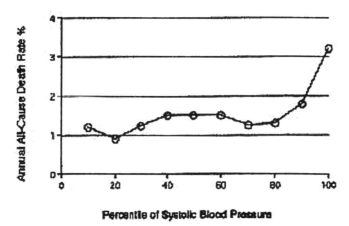

FIGURE 3.

FRAMINGHAM STUDY ALL-CAUSE DEATH RATES VS. PERCENTILE OF SYSTOLIC BLOOD PRESSURE FOR MEN AGED 45-74 YEARS. ADAPTED FROM PORT ET AL.[2]

With a better fit now, you see that if you are going to treat anyone for high blood pressure, you should treat only the top 10% of people, the 90th percentile. Everyone else is about equal.

TABLE 3.

SYSTOLIC BLOOD PRESSURE IN MM HG DEFINING THE 90TH PERCENTILE. THE LOWEST BP FOR WHICH MEDICAL TREATMENT IS JUSTIFIED.

Age	Female	Male
45-54	165	159
55-64	183	173
65-74	190	184

This table says that I, a 62 year old man, should be treated for high blood pressure only if my systolic blood pressure exceeds 173.

Mind, you still don't know whether treating the top 10% for high blood pressure will do any good; that fact can be determined only by doing an adequate randomized controlled trial. But at least you know not to bother with the lower 90% because the Framingham data shows that their morbidity is unrelated to blood pressure.

So the doctors blew it on the kick-off, but they haven't been sitting on their hands since then. They've been doing more studies, paid for by the pharmaceutical companies. Let's see what they saw when they used medicines to reduce the blood pressure in average people. I say "average" because–let's face it–that's what their study subjects were. Let's see how well that worked out.

TABLE 4.

A META-ANALYSIS OF STUDIES OF THE EFFECT OF ANTIHYPERTENSIVES ON PREVENTING STROKE, HEART ATTACK OR DEATH. DATA ARE % SURVIVORS. ARR=ABSOLUTE RISK REDUCTION, RRR= RELATIVE RISK REDUCTION.

	No. of studies	Drug	Control	ARR	RRR
Stroke					
Diuretics, high dose	9	98.9%	98.1%	0.8%	51±10%
Diuretics, low dose	4	95.6%	93.2%	2.4%	34±12%
Beta blockers	4	97.8%	97.2%	0.6%	29±12%
Heart disease					
Diuretics, high dose	11	97.3%	97.3%	0.0%	1±17%
Diuretics, low dose	4	95.0%	92.9%	2.1%	28± 8%
Beta-blockers	4	96.4%	96.2%	0.2%	7±13%
Mortality					
Diuretics, high dose	11	97.1%	96.8%	0.3%	12± 7%
Diuretics, low dose	4	88.1%	86.1%	2.0%	10± 9%
Beta-blockers	4	94.3%	94.2%	0.1%	5 ±11%

The original table was in the 2001 Kaplan *Textbook of Medicine*, page 973. The *relative risk reductions* were in the original table without the *absolute risk reductions*, but Joel Kauffman looked up the original articles and calculated the absolute risk reductions. I looked up the Medical Research Council trials and confirmed Joel's calculations.

Harking back to the discussion of relative and absolute risk reductions in Chapter 2, you know to discard the relative risk reductions. We are not insurance agents; relative risk reduction does not interest us.

Look at the absolute risk reductions instead. All pretty slim, eh? Joel thought it was a push, but I was ready to believe that low-dose diuretics were still marginally effective. The absolute risk reductions for strokes, heart attacks and death were all about 2%. Diuretics are cheap. I might pay 25 cents a day to reduce my chance of death by 2%.

But then I remembered that getting extra sodium in the diet in the 2011 Stolarz study reduced the absolute risk of death by 3.3% with a p=0.001%. My confidence in diuretics faded. How can it be that a diuretic, which makes you excrete sodium, and eating extra salt can both reduce your absolute risk of death? It can't be. One of the two facts must be wrong. I pick the diuretic to be wrong. I can't argue with a p value of 0.001 for sodium. (At this point I adjourn to eat a potato chip.)

Many studies and so much work have shown that reducing blood pressure with diuretics or beta blockers does not reduce heart attacks, strokes or death. Grasping at straws, you ask whether reducing blood pressure with newer drugs might work. Alas, the ALLHAT trial 2002 said no.[3] In that large study angiotensin-converting enzyme inhibitors and calcium channel blockers were compared to a simple diuretic. The diuretic out-performed both of the newer drugs. It was in all the newspapers. How did the pharmaceutical company sponsoring the ALLHAT trial let that truth slip out!

In summer of 2012 the prestigious Cochrane Review, the standard for evidence-based medicine, declared,

Antihypertensive drugs used in the treatment of adults (primary prevention) with mild hypertension (systolic BP 140-159 mmHg and/or diastolic BP 90-99 mmHg) have not been shown to reduce mortality or morbidity in randomized controlled trials.

What to do now?

If you are in the top 10% of the population for high blood pressure, you may reasonably take a blood pressure medicine to reduce your risk for stroke, heart attack or death. It won't make a big difference, but it might help a little. Don't take an expensive drug though. A cheap drug will do fine.

If you are not in the top 10%, there is no evidence that reducing your blood pressure will do anything useful.

I am supposed to tell you *not* to follow my advice without consulting your doctor. So I do say that. I say, *talk to your doctor*. But after you have listened to them, if they disagree with me, ask them one thing. Have they ever heard of Sid Port?

References

1. Port S Demer L Jennrich R et al. Systolic blood pressure and mortality. *Lancet* 2000;355:T175-180
2. Port S Garfinkle Boyle N. There is a non-linear relationship between mortality and blood pressure. *Euro Heart J* 2000;21:1635-1638.
3. ALLHAT trial. Major outcomes in high-risk hypertensive patients randomized to angiotensin-converting enzyme inhibitor or calcium channel blocker vs. diuretic. *JAMA* 2002;288:2981-2997
4. Stolarz-Skrzypek K, Kuznetsova T, Thijs L et al. Fatal and non-fatal outcomes, incidence of hypertension and blood pressure changes in relation to urinary sodium excretion. *JAMA* 2011;305:1777-1785.

MYTH #5

High cholesterol causes heart attacks.

Fact

Nope. And lowering cholesterol doesn't prevent them either, unless you have a rare genetic disease called familial hypercholesterolemia, and even then, maybe not.

Why we should have known better

Cholesterol is an essential cell component in animal tissues. Is it likely that raising the blood level of cholesterol a little, say from 199 mg/dl to 240 mg/dl, would cause a disease? Can you name any other situation in which raising the level of a normal body constituent so little causes an illness? No and no.

Lowering cholesterol with drugs has not reduced the number of heart attacks per 100,000 people in the U.S. This statement will surprise most physicians, used to hearing that their wholesale prescription of statin drugs has reduced the incidence of heart attacks. Consider the passage below from the CDC website http://www.cdc.gov/mmwr/ preview/ mmwrhtml/mm4830a1.htm. Among the "Factors Contributing to the Decline in CVD Deaths" the article correctly cites the reduction in smoking since 1950 and improvements in acute medical care at hospitals, but then the article goes on to list the following as causes for the reduction in heart attack deaths:

- a decrease in mean blood pressure levels in the U.S. population (11,13,14). an increase in the percentage of persons with hypertension who have the condition treated and controlled. **I showed you in the previous Myth that this idea is wrong.**

- a decrease in mean blood cholesterol levels and changes in the U.S. diet. Data based on surveys of food supply suggest that consumption of saturated fat and cholesterol has decreased since 1909. Data from the National Health and Nutrition Examination surveys suggest that decreases in the percentage of calories from dietary fat and the levels of dietary cholesterol coincide with decreases in blood cholesterol levels. **I will now show you that this is a Myth also.**

In fact, the incidence of heart attacks has declined all over the world since 1950, even in countries with no access to statin drugs. It has declined even in countries that don't, and never did, eat much fat in the diet.

By the time the statin drugs arrived in the U.S. in 1987, the dramatic reduction in heart attacks had already occurred. Look at the time-line in the next figure.

USA death rates for major cardiovascular diseases 1900-2007

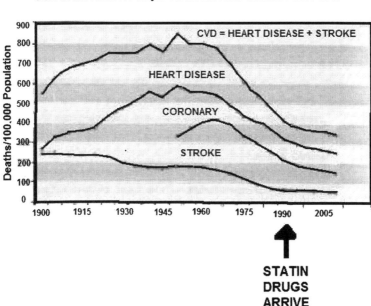

While *mortality* from heart attacks continued to decline through the nineties in the U.S., the overall *number* of heart attacks per 100,000 people has stayed about the same. The small amount of reduction that may have occurred is attributable to the removal of trans fats from the food supply and the reduction in psychosocial stress. I have to prove all this, of course, and I will.

How we got confused
By putting too much faith in epidemiological comparisons, not doing enough good comparisons, and waiting too long to do proper prospective trials. And the old problem, looking at relative risk reduction instead of absolute risk reduction.

Once the cholesterol hypothesis appeared, we stopped pursuing alternative ideas. A fourth of every research budget should go to skeptics, because . . .

All progress comes not from trying to prove what we believe is true, but from trying to disprove it.
                    Francis Bacon, the inventor of scientific method

How did the Cholesterol Hypothesis get started? First, a man named Virchow, doing autopsies on patients who had died from heart attack, noticed that in the blood clots in the blocked coronary arteries there were crystals identifiable as cholesterol. His observation was correct, but not so interesting–there is cholesterol in all blood clots. LDL, the particle in blood carrying cholesterol, sticks to fibrin, the protein of blood clots. Virchow did not say the cholesterol he saw *caused* the atherosclerosis; he was too good a scientist to confuse association with cause. Unfortunately, many doctors since Virchow's time were not so careful.

Other doctors later assumed that cholesterol was an essential feature of atherosclerotic blood vessels, even the cause of them; and that if you could reduce the cholesterol in blood, you would prevent heart attacks and strokes. A defining moment came in 1953 when Ancel Keys presented the Seven Countries Study.

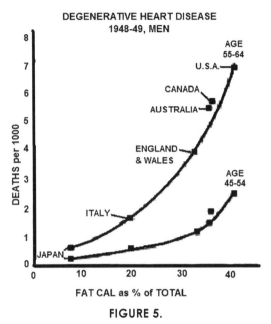

FIGURE 5.

THE SEVEN COUNTRIES STUDY, ANCEL KEYS 1953

When Keys made a graph of the amount of fat in the diet on the X-axis and heart attacks on the Y-axis, he found that seven countries fell nicely along a rising curve. The countries with the least fat in the diet, Japan and Italy, had the fewest heart attacks. The countries with the most fat in the diet, the U.S. and Canada, had the most.

After that study, dietitians began to recommend that the American public eat less fat. The public responded. They substituted sugar for fat. Following that, *and as a result of that mistake*, diabetes, obesity, heart attacks and gallstones took off in the U.S.

Keys made the same calculations for other countries, but did not include the data in his graph. For example, he did not include France. He didn't say why, but I know why.

France does not not fall on the nice curve. The French point is way off the line in the lower right hand corner.

Moreover, since the Seven Countries study was done, the cardiac death rates of all seven countries have strayed all over the map. They would not fit on any smooth curve today!

Look at the map of Europe below.

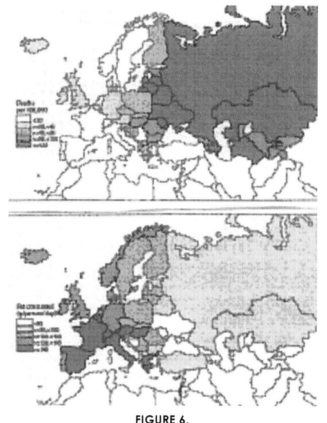

FIGURE 6.

EUROPE. TOP. PREVALENCE OF HEART ATTACKS. ORANGE MEANS HIGH.
BOTTOM. FAT CONSUMPTION PER CAPITA.

The upper panel shows that the mortality from heart attacks and strokes is highest in eastern Europe. The lower panel shows that the people in western Europe eat more fat. The two distributions could not be more different![2] How could anyone believe fat causes heart attacks?

But the genie was out of the bottle. The pharmaceutical companies had identified a target, cholesterol, and there would be more targets to follow: saturated fat, LDL, HDL, triglycerides to name a few. Each promised rich rewards for the pharmaceutical companies and the doctors working for them.

I became a doctor in the early seventies in the midst of the feeding frenzy. I remember the haste and the money flying around. When the first statin drug, Mevacor (lovastatin) reached the market, doctors thought the "cholesterol problem" had been solved, never mind that there was never a cholesterol problem in the first place . . .

Except with the few people with a rare genetic disorder called familial hypercholesterolemia (FHC). They don't have cholesterols of 250 or 280. They have numbers like 400, 600, and they may, indeed, get more heart attacks. Even that is not certain since the only way people with FHC get into the medical system is by having a heart attack or getting their cholesterol checked. No one knows how many people with FHC are out wandering about, refusing to get a heart attack or a test. If cholesterol really is a problem for the FHC people, then statin drugs may be good for them.

Maybe, but the statin drugs also reduce the synthesis of coenzyme Q-10, dolichol, sex hormones and nuclear factor kappa B. I'll get to all that later.

As Kai Ryssdal says on *Marketplace*, let's do the numbers! using almost the same format as before in Myth #5. Here are the major statin trials with their relative and absolute risk reductions. Since the trials had different lengths, we have to divide the absolute risk reductions by the number of years in the trial in order to compare the trials. First we focus on all-cause mortality.

TABLE 5.

RANDOMIZED CONTROLLED TRIALS ON THE EFFECT OF STATINS ON ALL-CAUSE MORTALITY. LOOK FOR THE ABSOLUTE RISK REDUCTION (ARR) PER YEAR. A + SIGN MEANS THE STATIN WAS ASSOCIATED WITH *MORE* DEATH. A - SIGN MEANS LESS DEATH.

Study	Drug Used	Years	RRR	ARR	ARR/year
EXCEL	Mevacor	1	+150%	+0.3%	+0.30%
AFCAPS	Mevacor	5.2	+ 3.9%	+0.1%	+0.02%
4S	Zocor	5.4	-29%	-3.3%	-0.61%
HPS	Zocor	5.0	-12%	-1.8%	-0.36%
WOSCOPS	Pravachol	4.4	-22%	-0.9%	-0.20%
PROSPER	Pravachol	3.1	-1.9%	-0.2%	-0.07%
LIPID	Pravachol	6.1	-22%	-3.1%	-0.51%
CARE	Pravachol	5.0	- 8%	-0.8%	-0.15%
ALLHAT-LLT	Pravachol	6.0	zero	-0.6%	-0.10%
ASCOT	Lipitor	3.3	-12%	-0.5%	-0.15%
JUPITER	Crestor	5.0	-20%	-0.4%	-0.08%

From Kauffman *Malignant Medical Myths*, page 89.

RRR = relative risk reduction. AAR = absolute risk reduction.

The absolute risk reductions ranged from +0.3% to -3.3%. Surely a negative result. So the statin drugs don't prevent the worst heart attacks, the ones that kill right away. But maybe they prevent *non-fatal* heart attacks, like the one I had in 2004. Look at Table 6. There is a little surprise at the end.

TABLE 6.

RANDOMIZED CONTROLLED TRIALS ON THE PREVENTION
OF NON-FATAL HEART ATTACKS

Study	Drug Used	Years	RR	ARR	ARR/year
AFCAPS	Mevacor	5.2	-38%	-2.0%	-0.38%
4S	Zocor	5.4	-30%	-6.7%	-1.24%
WOSCOPS	Pravachol	4.4	-22%	-1.8%	-0.41%
PROSPER	Pravachol	3.1	-12%	-1.0%	-0.32%
LIPID	Pravachol	6.1	-27%	-2.9%	-0.48%
CARE	Pravachol	5.0	-22%	-1.8%	-0.36%
ALLHAT-LLT	Pravachol	6.0	- 2%	-0.1%	-0.02%
ASCOT	Lipitor	3.3	-37%	-1.1%	-0.33%
PHS	buffered aspirin	7.0	-59%	-0.76	-0.76%

From Kauffman *Malignant Medical Myths* page 93.

The statins were no better at preventing non-fatal heart attacks either, with one exception, the 4S Trial, which I will discuss below.

The surprise I mentioned was that we included aspirin at the end of the table to show that a measly cheap *buffered* aspirin works better than the statin drugs at preventing heart attacks. But don't get too worked up over it. Studies using *plain* aspirin showed no benefit. It may be that the magnesium in buffered aspirin is responsible for the benefit seen in the PHS trial. More about that later.

None of the statin absolute risk reductions were over 1% except the 4S trial. That trial contained patients who had already had one heart attack. It was what we call a "secondary prevention" trial. In that setting there was, indeed, some protection from a second heart attack.

Now get this. *The statin protection from heart attack, what little we see, is unrelated to the degree of reduction in cholesterol.* The protective effect, seen in trials like the 4S, does not come from reducing cholesterol. That's no surprise to you because I taught you that cholesterol has nothing to do with heart attacks. Indeed, 75% of the heart attacks occurring today occur in people whose cholesterol meets the current ATP 3 guidelines. http://www.sciencedaily.com/releases/2009/01/090112130653.htm. That's because doctors have gotten the cholesterol levels down and still the heart attacks go on.

The new thinking is that statin drugs work as an anti-inflammatory The plaques in the walls of the arteries, the ones that rupture http://en.wikipedia.org/wiki/ JUPITER_trial. re, are often *inflamed*, infiltrated with white blood cells, like a sore on the skin. No one really knows why they are inflamed. There was some excitement over the idea that the plaques were infected by bacteria, but that idea has faded. The c-reactive protein or hsCRP test gives some indication of the degree of inflammation.

The mechanism of the anti-inflammatory effect is that statins reduce nuclear factor kappa B (NF-kB), a transcription factor that prepares white blood cells to fight germs or cancer.[5] That's good in a way–inflammation in the artery wall does no one any good. But in another way, it's bad because your body is less able to fight small cancers, allowing them to grow into big cancers. An important job of the immune system is to kill microscopic cancers.

Statins kill people in other ways besides allowing cancer to grow. Statins cause congestive heart failure, or make it worse, by making the heart pump more weakly.[5,6] You already knew that statins made your arm and leg muscles hurt; statin drugs affect the heart muscle, too.

Statins increase the incidence of depression. In large studies more statin patients died from suicide and from accidental and violent deaths, all probably related to depression[5]. In April 2012 the FDA ordered the makers of statin drugs to include warnings that the drugs impair memory and cause or worsen diabetes.

What to do now?

No one should take a statin drug except . . .

- for a short period of time after a first heart attack, to prevent a second heart attack. I'm not sure how long the protective effect lasts.
- People with familial hypercholesterolemia should take a statin. Maybe. It depends. We're not sure.

I am supposed to tell you to talk to your doctor and follow their advice. So I say it–talk to your doctor. But if he or she shows no sign of knowing about absolute risk reduction, you should buy him or her a copy of my book. If they show no curiosity about that either, you should find a new doctor.

References

1. Keys A. Seven countries: a multivariate analysis of death and coronary heart disease. London: Harvard University Press, 1980.
2. Kendrick talking to the British Medical Association http://www.youtube.com/watch?v=XPPYaVcXo1I
3. Kauffman J. *Malignant Medical Myths*. Infinity Publishing, 2006.
4. Kendrick M. *The Great Cholesterol Con*. John Blake Publishing, London, 2008
5. Graveline D. *The Statin Damage Crisis. 2006*
6. Rubinstein J Aloka F Abela GS. Statin therapy decreases myocardial function as evaluated via strain imaging. *Clin Cardiol* 2009;32:684-689.

MYTH #6

High blood sugar causes heart attacks.

Fact

Not so.

Why we should have known better

For you to understand the evidence, I must teach you three facts about diabetes.

1. There are two types of diabetes. Type 1 is the least common, about 10% of all diabetics. In type 1 the cells in the pancreas that produce insulin have been wiped out. Since insulin is necessary to move glucose (sugar) from the blood into the tissues, type 1 patients are dependent on insulin shots to live.
2. Patients with type 2 diabetes make plenty of insulin. But they eat so much that their pancreas can't keep up–they can't make enough insulin. And their tissues are resistant to insulin.
3. Doctors keep track of the average blood sugar over time by measuring the HbA_{1c} or hemoglobin A_{1c}.

Now here is the evidence. The Pittsburgh Epidemiology of Diabetes Complications Study reported *no association* between HbA_{1c} and the 4-year incidence of heart attacks; that means no association between the average blood sugar and heart attacks.[1] Moreover, in the large Diabetes Control and Complications Trial , intensive insulin therapy, to keep the blood sugar at consistent low levels, did not reduce the incidence of major cardiovascular events.[2,3,4]

None of the type 1 diabetic patients I ever saw in my practice–they were all lean–showed any sign of large vessel atherosclerosis, though they did have problems with their eyes, nerves and kidneys. Good control helped with those things, just not with heart attacks.

How we got confused

We got confused because type 2 diabetics *do* get more heart attacks. The incidence of heart attacks increases with the HbA_{1c} or blood sugar in type 2 diabetics in many large studies. The association is present even after adjusting for gender, smoking, weight, blood pressure, and cholesterol.

So you might think better control of blood sugar in type 2 diabetics would lead to fewer heart attacks, but it does not. In the UKPDS Trial control of blood sugar with insulin or an oral drug did not significantly reduce heart attacks.[5] The issue is not as clear as for type 1 diabetes, because good comprehensive care of type 2 diabetics, restraining their consumption of carbs and getting them to lose weight, does reduce heart attacks. But therapy focused entirely on the blood sugar does nothing. So you have to say that high blood sugar itself does not cause heart attacks.

What to do now?

Diabetics, please, get control of your blood sugar, but not because you believe doing so will prevent a heart attack. Do it because it will preserve your nerves, eyes and kidneys.

References

1. Orchard TJ: From diagnosis and classification to complications and therapy. DCCT Part II? The 1993 Kelly West Lecture. *Diabetes Care* 1994;17:326-328.
2. Kuusisto J Mykkanen L Pyorala K Laakso M. NIDDM and its metabolic control predict coronary artery disease in elderly subjects. *Diabetes* 1994;43:960-967.
3. Singer DE Nathan DM Anderson KM et al. Association of HBA1c with prevalent cardiovascular diseas in

the original cohort of the Framingham Heart Study. *Diabetes* 1992;41:202-208.

4. Wei M Gaskill SP Haffner SM Stern MP. Effects of diabetes and level of glycemia on all-cause and cardiovascular mortality. *Diabetes Care* 1998;21:1167-1172.

5. UK Prospective Diabetes Study (UKPDS) Group. Intensive blood-glucose control with sulphonylureas or insulin compared with conventional treatment and risk of complications in patients with type 2 diabetes. *Lancet* 1998;352:837-853.

BRIEF INTERRUPTION

If you've made it this far in this book, you may be thinking, Dr. Anchors seems opposed to everything. You think, the situation can't be that bad. So many smart doctors, with white coats and nice offices, working together, could not have gotten so much wrong.

Why not? A lot of smart college grads in the Middle Ages worked together to come up with the theory that the flat Earth was the center of the universe. They got that wrong. The smart economists and business leaders who brought us the financial meltdown of 2008 were smart, too.

I laugh, you see, because if I was talking about incompetence in the federal government, most Americans would not blink an eye. Americans scorn their elected officials, but they love the guys in white coats who write their prescriptions. If the patients still get heart attacks and cancer, it can't be the doctor's fault, right? Americans have loved their doctors from the days of Dr. Kildare and Marcus Welby down to Dr. Phil and Dr. Oz.

I AGREE doctors can't get everything wrong all the time. That is why there is a section in the back of this book on the things doctors got right.

But doctors allow themselves to be misled by the pharmaceutical companies. Doctors prescribe so many expensive medicines that do not work. They give medicines for things that don't need to be treated.

Don't go squishy soft on me, now when we are just getting started. There are more myths to tackle.

I am passionate about my subject because the refusal of American doctors to think on their own or challenge the propaganda from the pharmaceutical companies has made medicine in the U.S. so much more expensive, and often less effective, than medicine in Europe. The U.S. spends $5635 per person per year on health care. The European Union countries spend $2572, and get better results. Click on http://www.mckinsey.com/mgi/publications/healthcare/slideshow/interactive.asp.

The U.S. is the only developed nation in the world that does not have a single payer system, i.e. either socialized medicine or national health insurance. We could join the civilized world in having a better system, but we are blocked by the unnecessary high cost of health care in America. The chief source of the expense is the persistence of doctors in prescribing medicines that don't work or aren't necessary.

This is the Hippocratic Oath taken by most new doctors at the time of graduation from medical school. Do doctors keep their oath?

"I SWEAR in the presence of the Almighty and before my family, my teachers and my peers that according to my ability and judgment I will keep this Oath and Stipulation.

"TO RECKON all who have taught me this art equally dear to me as my parents and in the same spirit and dedication to impart a knowledge of the art of medicine to others. **I will continue with diligence to keep abreast of advances in medicine.** I will treat without exception all who seek my ministrations, so long as the treatment of others is not compromised thereby, **and I will seek the counsel of**

particularly skilled physicians where indicated for the benefit of my patient.

"I WILL FOLLOW that method of treatment which according to my ability and judgment, I consider for the benefit of my patient and abstain from whatever is harmful or mischievous."

Do you think most doctors keep their oath? Does listening to the verbal representations of the drug company reps or reading their written propaganda suffice for "keeping abreast with advances in medicine"? Is everything new an advance? Or do you expect doctors to read original studies, go behind the scenes, talk to true experts and think deeply about medicine. The following is a letter written by a doctor in censoring the speech I was going to give at a public institution.

"I have reviewed Dr. Anchors' lecture notes and have decided not to sponsor his lecture. My reasoning is this–although I agree with much of his discussion, his interpretation of the data on a few important points is in the minority among medical scientists.

"When reviewing an employee's health and risk factors during the annual physical exam, I advise him or her on health risks. Not being in a position to do research or directly interpret research data, I rely on the written opinion of scientists who do

"Although it is not unusual to get a difference of opinion on some medical science issues, still a consensus for recommendations is reached, and I adhere to those. Dr. Anchors is opposed to that consensus on some issues, and could bring confusion to some of our folks.

Dr. B."

I can only observe that Freedom of Speech is useless without the Freedom to Hear!

Now here is an e-mail from a teenager in New York City.

"I just put down a copy of Medical Myths, which I found on a coffee table while visiting a family friend. After reading the first chapter I couldn't put it down, and proceeded to skim the entire volume. I found the book fascinating, informative and terrifying, and I would love to have my own copy as well as a copy to send to my father (a doctor).

"I want to let you know that I think this is an extremely important book. As you've demonstrated, too much information in the medical industry, and more generally the United States, is taken at face value. As a college student and aspiring intellectual, I'm beginning to understand the importance of questioning facts and independently evaluating data. I'm not personally interested in the medical fields, but I am interested in learning to think. Your book is a beautiful demonstration of critical investigation. Thank you so much for taking the time to articulate your knowledge, and I hope this book finds its way onto every shelf in the US.

"Please let me know how to obtain copies of the book.
"Thank you,
L. A."

Tell me, who is the better doctor? Dr. B or the young woman in New York?

MYTH #7

The food pyramids from the U.S. Department of Agriculture, used by nutritionists and taught in schools.[1]

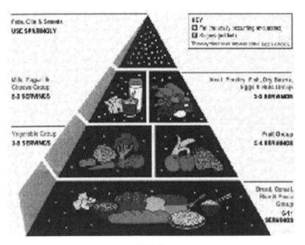

FIG.7.

THE UPSIDE-DOWN PYRAMID FROM 1992

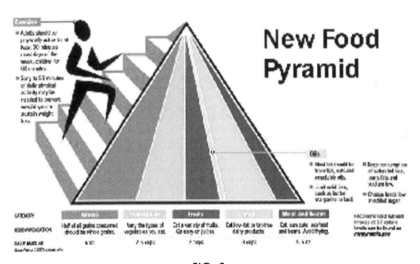

FIG. 8.

THE MEANINGLESS THING FROM 2005

Fact

Here is the correct food pyramid, published by Dr. Anchors in 1997 as part of his phen-pro weight-loss program,[3] and often used now by nutritionists following their own experience as a guide.

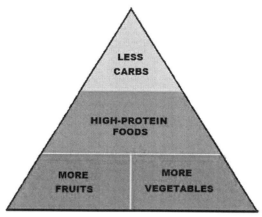

FIG. 9.

DR. ANCHORS' FOOD PYRAMID, THE CORRECT FOOD PYRAMID

Why we should have known better

Who expects the Department of Agriculture to be experts on healthy diet? You expect such information to come from the CDC or the Department of Health, not from the department charged with protecting U.S. farmers. The USDA didn't even do the 2005 Pyramid itself; they hired the Porter-Novelli Company to do it.[4] Porter Novelli is a Washington-based PR firm whose clients include Mountain Dew soda. Take out your telescope and see if you can spot a conflict of interest there.

OF COURSE the USDA and Porter-Novelli tell you to eat lots of corn! The U.S. with only 4.7% of the world's population produces 30% of the world's crop.[2] The USDA wants to move the stuff off the farm. But does that mean that eating so much corn is good for you, or for the cattle and chickens?

It isn't. Read *The Omnivore's Dilemma* by Michael Pollan (Penguin Press, 2006), or shucks! I will explain it all below.

How we got confused

The initial source of confusion was this. Fat has 9 calories/per gram. Carbohydrates and protein have only 3-4 calories/ gram. Obese people take in more calories than they spend in activity. So without any other knowledge, if you were going to pick on a food group for having too many calories, the obvious target would be fat.

But wait, you need more knowledge. Eat all the fat you want and all the carbs and protein–you won't store much *unless the blood level of insulin is high*. The hormone insulin, from the pancreas, is the switch that tells your body to store energy. If the switch is off, little fat gets stored, no matter what you eat.

Even though dietary fat is rich in calories, it is a poor stimulus to insulin. The stimulus that really sets insulin off is carbohydrate.

- That is why you don't store fat unless you eat carbs with it.
- That is why type I diabetics are initially lean. They can't make insulin, so they can't store fat. They can't store fat until the doctor puts them on insulin shots.
- That is why obese people developing type 2 diabetes initially lose weight. Their gross overeating of carbs finally outruns their ability to make insulin.

The carbohydrates in fruits and vegetables, especially uncooked or undercooked vegetables, are a medium-strong stimulus to insulin. The human body has been seeing these food items for a million years–it's used to them.

But the "bad carbs", table sugar and and high-fructose corn syrup (HFCS), are new to the Earth. They are a strong stimulus to insulin. The human body has not adapted to them.

Table sugar was brought to us by Christopher Columbus, and HFCS by Richard Nixon. Columbus killed more people than any other human in history. Perhaps I should explain.

About the time Columbus discovered America, the Portuguese discovered sugar cane in Indonesia. The Europeans transplanted sugar cane from Indonesia to the Caribbean islands where it grew taller and thicker than in its original home. That was the first time Europeans had a rich, pure source of sucrose.

At first they shipped sugar back to Europe as rum since sugar itself tended to spoil in the ships. Rum was the first distilled spirit. Before that, all the Europeans had was wine and beer. They liked rum!

Eventually Europeans perfected the skill of getting sugar itself back to Europe. Before that, all they had to sweeten food was honey. They preferred sugar! Within a generation the obesity rate of Europeans shot up. King Henry VIII, Charles V, Pope Leo X and Suleiman the Magnificent (Turkey) were rotund, and they had diabetes and gout.

Along with sugar and rum going back to the Old World was tobacco and syphilis, a lethal harvest that killed many Europeans.

But the Europeans had it good compared to the Native Americans. Their legacy from Columbus was small pox, hepatitis and racial slavery. By the time the English colonists moved westward, they moved into what seemed like virgin forest. It wasn't virgin. 70% of the native Americans had died ahead of them. Read *1491* by Charles Mann (Vintage Books, 2006).

Now about Richard Nixon . . .

Starting after the New Deal, the U.S. government had a program of lending money to farmers at planting time at low interest, collecting money back after the harvest. Some crops received price supports, so that if the market price fell too low, the federal government would buy grain from farmers and store it in the national grain reserve. These wise policies stabilized food prices and permitted U.S. farmers to lead a more comfortable life.

In the early seventies the Soviet Union had several poor harvests and famine threatened. Nixon, wishing to improve relations with the Soviet Union, sold them most of the U.S. grain reserve at low prices. He sold so much grain that the price of food in the U.S. shot up dramatically, just before the midterm elections.

Nixon afraid the Republicans would lose the election, instructed Secretary of Agriculture Earl "Rusty" Butts to do anything necessary to get the price of food down quickly. Rusty instituted the policy of paying American farmers directly to grow corn. If they wanted to grow cucumbers, they could get a loan, but if they would grow corn, they got straight cash.

Why corn? because corn provides more calories per acre than any other crop. Granted you have to use a lot of petroleum-based fertilizers to do this, but hey! the election was at stake.

The trick worked; food prices fell. The GOP did okay in the election. After that, came Watergate, and the rest is his-story. But the strange thing is that, in 2011, 38 years after Nixon, we are still paying farmers to grow corn, specifically. We grow far more than we need. We don't export much. We feed the stuff to our cows and chickens who had never seen corn before. We keep the beasts alive with antibiotics, slaughter them young and eat 'em. It's all in Michael Pollan's book.

The federal deficit is now 14 trillion dollars; Americans are obese; we are looking for places to cut federal expenditures, and yet, we are still paying farmers directly to grow corn. I have an idea . . .

What to do now?

Stop paying farmers to grow any particular crop not in short supply. Let the price of food rise to its equilibrium market value. If the objection is that poor people will be harmed, let them eat less food. America is the first nation in the world to have obese poor people. Offer food stamps and other supports only to people not grossly overweight.

The CDC should produce a truthful food pyramid. It will, of course, be my pyramid. The USDA should get out of the business of producing food pyramids altogether and stick to its core area of competency.

BULLETIN! Literally as I was typing this, June 2, 2011, Michelle Obama announced that the USDA (and Porter Novelli) was substituting the new MyPlate icon for the old, failed 2005 MyPyramid.

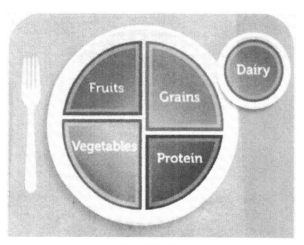

FIGURE 10.
MyPlate.com

Just the old, discredited five food groups from 1954 repackaged as a colorful circle. Shame. Why didn't they talk to any scientists?

References

1. http://www.disabled-world.com/artman/publish/food_pyramid.shtml
2. http://www.indexmundi.com/agriculture/?commodity=corn&graph=production
3. Anchors M. Update on the phen-pro combination and my views on obesity in America. *The Bariatrician*

Fall 2002, page 17 - 22, and two published books *Safer Than Phen-fen* (Prima, 1997) and *Life Between Meals* (Anchors Books, 2006).

4. http://www.porternovelli.com/offerings/

MYTH #8

The BMI or body mass index is the best way to tell if you are obese.

Fact

Not so.

Why we should have known better

The BMI was never intended to be used for individual people; it was invented as a tool for population studies.[1] It ignores body shape and composition. According to the BMI the two people shown below would have the same risks if their weight and height were the same.

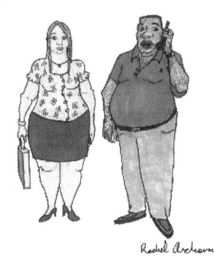

FIG. 11

We know they don't. The man on the right is at a much greater risk of heart attack, diabetes and death because of his apple shape.[2]

How we got confused

Let me take you back to 1998. The dangers of fenfluramine, the bad half of phen-fen, had just been exposed. Doctors who had prescribed fenfluramine were in danger of being sued for malpractice, particularly if they had prescribed fenfluramine to patients who were not technically obese.

But what did "obese" mean? No formal body had defined it. The lawyers wanted a universal definition so they could prosecute doctors. Pharmaceutical companies wanted a definition to give doctors guidance on when to prescribe diet drugs. The FDA wanted a definition.

A medical conference was convened.[3] The fix was in from the moment the panel opened. It had already been decided by the conference leaders that the BMI would be used, for one simple reason. The BMI required only the weight and height to calculate, and every doctor already had those measurements on the patient's chart. The leaders wanted something NOW, not necessarily something right.,

Everyone knew waist size or body fat percentage would be a better parameter, but few practicing doctors had measured those items. The panel needed something immediately because doctors were in imminent danger of being sued for their *past* behavior. The doctors in court could use only what they had actually measured.

The BMI equals the weight W in kilograms divided by the square of the height H in meters. Using pounds and inches instead of kilograms and meters, you have to multiply the whole shebang by 703.

$$BMI = \frac{703 \times W}{H^2}$$

The panel decided that a BMI of 25 would be the upper limit of normal. The territory between 25 and 30 would be called "overweight", and the region above 30 would be called "obese". BMI over 40 would be called "morbidly obese". All of these were strange new usages of the words. Before that "overweight" just meant being over someone's idea of how much you should weigh. The reason for overweight wasn't specified. You could be overweight if you had too much fat, too much muscle or too much change in your pockets.

The word "obese" was a straight borrowing from a Latin word meaning 'too fat'. But how much was too much? And where? It was known that visceral fat, the fat around the gut, played a greater role in heart attacks than the fat underneath skin or in the buttocks and legs.

"Morbidly" was a strange choice, because it implied that only obesity of the fifth dimension was sufficient to cause death, when everyone knew that BMI in the 30-40 range also contributed to death.

The choice of 25 and 30 as the cutoff points was suspicious. Such neat, round numbers. Do you suppose they were drawn from real studies of Nature, which is usually anything but neat?

Indeed, two years after the consensus conference Bill Dietz at the CDC had shown that the risk of type 2 diabetes is already doubled at a BMI of 23.[4] Perhaps 22 should have been chosen as the dividing point.

There was nothing magic about the 30 mark either. The risk of heart attack and death increases smoothly upward at every BMI over 22. Why call a person with a BMI of 29 "normal" and a person with BMI 31 "obese" when their risks are so similar?

What to do now?

Leave the BMI to the epidemiologists who invented it. Stop using it to make decisions on individual people. Use the waist size instead, or just look at people. If their abdomen is bursting out over their belt, you don't need a statistical parameter to tell they are fat and in danger. If the doctor's word on this is not good enough in court, then what have we come to?

References

1. Dyer AR Stamler J Berkson DM et al. Relationship of relative weight and body mass index to 14 year mortality in the Chicago Peoples Gas Company Study. *J Chronic Dis* 1975;28:109-123.
2. Rexrode KM Carey VJ Hennekens CH et al. Abdominal adiposity and coronary heart disease. *JAMA* 1998;280:1843-1848.
3. Clinical guidelines on the identification, evaluation and treament of overweight and obesity in adults: executive summary. Expert Panel on the Identification and Treatment of Overweight in Adults. *Am J Clin Nutr* 1998;68:899-917.
4. Field AE Coakley EH Must A et al. Impact of overweight on the risk of developing common chronic diseases during a 10-year period. *Arch Int Med* 2001;161:1581-1586.

MYTH #9

Strenuous exercise is good for you.

Fact

Moderate exercise is good for you. Strenuous exercise is more likely to leave you injured or dead.

Why we should have known better

When Pheidippides finished the first marathon run in 490 BCE carrying the news of the Greek victory over the Persians, he dropped dead. The same fate befell Jim Fixx, author of *The Complete Book of Running*. In fact on average, runners live *less* long than non-runners.[1]   And 20% of men running 30 miles a week and 25% of women have an injury requiring a visit to the doctor [2]

How we got confused
By putting blind faith in testimonials and anecdotes and never reading the actual data with an objective view. Most people, *even the authors of studies*, believe that exercise makes you healthier and the more the better. They don't even notice when their own data contradicts them.

For instance, in a study by Jakecic, principally a study of losing weight, obese subjects were instructed in a balanced low-calorie diet (the DASH diet) and then randomized to four groups.[3] One group did heavy exercise on a treadmill for a short period of time, another group heavy exercise for a long period, another light exercise for a short period for a long period. All four groups lost the same small amount of weight in a year, 10 lb average, but the authors still insisted in their summary that exercise was an effective adjunct to diet in helping people lose weight. They didn't look at their own data.

The Jakicic study didn't bother to include a no-exercise control group; the authors were so certain that exercise would help people lose weight that they focused only on trying to determine which type of exercise was best weight. They were half-way down the road before they remembered to check whether they were even on the right street.

Most of the people out jogging believe they are losing weight. You see them month after month, year after year, and they are always the same size! For them, seeing is not believing. Believing is believing. But in fact, exercise hardly helps fat people lose weight at all. There was a big spread on this topic in *TIME*, August 17, 2009, "Will exercise make you thin?" written by John Cloud. The author concluded that exercise would not make you thin.

Here is why. Because very fat people burn so many calories doing nothing, even lying still in bed. A 300 lb man has to pump a double blood volume. Breathing is difficult due to the thickness of the chest wall. The fat-filled abdomen pushes up against the diaphragm. Such people do not have to go to the gym to exercise. They ARE a gym. Indeed, going to the gym is only dangerous for them. They are at greater risk for orthopedic injuries and sudden death.

For lean people, on the other hand, exercise is not so dangerous. Exercise helps keep them lean.[4,5]

But all in moderation.

Some people are compulsive runners. They continue to run even when it is obvious they are giving themselves osteoporosis and arthritis. What do you call it when people persist in a behavior in the face of obvious adverse consequences? You call it "addiction". There is an extensive literature on the relationship between addiction and compulsive exercise.

In the current DSM-IV, the book defining psychiatric diagnoses, compulsive running has even been designated as a form of bulimia. I know it is correct because I have seen that the same medicine combination, phen-pro, tremendously helps both bulimia and compulsive running.

What to do now?

Stop over-exercising or under-exercising. America is the land of crazy extremes. Most people do either too much exercise or no exercise at all. Exercise should be scaled to body weight, gender and physical conditioning. The body of many a weekend warrior lies a'mouldering in the grave.

References

1. Dorn J Naughton J Imamura D et al. Results of a multicenter radnomized clinical trial of exercise and

long-term survival in Myocardial infarction patients. *Circulation* 1999;100:1764-1769.

2. Koplan JP Powell KE Sikes RK et al. An epidemiologic study of the benefits and risks of running. *JAMA* 1983;248:3118-3121.

3. Goodpaster BH DeLany JP Otto AD et al. Effects of diet and physical activity interventions on weight loss and cardiometabolic risk factors in severely obese adults. *JAMA* 2010;304:1795-1802.

4. Donnelly JE Hill JO Jacobsen DJ et al. Effects of a 16month randomized controlled exercise trial on body weight and composition in young, overweight men and women. *Arch Intern Med* 2003;163:1343-1350.

5. Hankinson AL Daviglus ML Bouchard C et al. Maintaining a high physical activity level over 20 years and weight gain. *JAMA* 2010;304:2603-2610.

MYTH #10

Diet pills are bad for you.

Fact

Fenfluramine, the "fen" in phen-fen or fen-phen (same thing), was indeed bad for you, but it's off the market now. Phentermine, the "phen" in phen-fen is still safe, and legal.[1,2,3,4] The trouble is that 60% of non-doctors and 99.9% of American doctors cannot tell a "fen" from a "phen". They have completely confused the two drugs.

Why we should have known better

Phentermine, 52 years old, is still safe and going strong.[5,6,7] Indeed, it's almost the only diet pill left. Millions of people have taken the medicine and lost weight with it. I know. I am the patent holder of the phen-pro combination, have written books and appeared on TV. I have been in the thick of the diet pill issue since 1995. You may take account of my bias on the issue, but you cannot doubt my experience.

How we got confused

Phentermine works, it reduces hunger, but it works for only about six weeks and then loses steam. Around 1992 Dr. Michael Weintraub discovered that if fenfluramine was added to phentermine, the combination of pills worked longer and better than either medicine alone.[8] Someone–I don't know who–called this combination the phen-fen combination, or sometimes fen-phen. I'd like to wring his neck because he confused everyone.

Fenfluramine was a new diet pill just coming to the U.S. from Switzerland. At the time it was thought to be an SSRI drug, i.e. a serotonin reuptake inhibitor like Prozac the famous antidepressant. I began giving phen-fen to patients, about a dozen, and had good success. But fenfluramine, also called Pondimin, was expensive. I reasoned that if fenfluramine worked like Prozac, why not use Prozac itself in the combination instead of fenfluramine? Prozac was cheaper.

The Phentermine/Prozac combination, dubbed "phen-pro" by other people (not by me!) worked as well as phen-fen. I stopped using phen-fen. I got the patent for phen-pro in 1998.[9]

So almost from the beginning, phen-pro coexisted with phen-fen. Phen-fen was like the big dinosaur. Phen-pro lived in the shadows like the mammals between the legs of the dinosaurs. Few doctors knew about it. Surprisingly so, since I published and appeared on radio, TV and in magazines, but we know that practicing doctors are a little out of touch.[10]

You know what happened to the dinosaurs; the same thing happened to phen-fen. A meteor hit the Earth in summer of 1997. Heidi Connolly and her colleagues at the Mayo

Clinic published that fenfluramine caused heart valve damage in a significant number of people.[11,12]

Well, that's what she should have said. What she did say, instead, was that *phen-fen* was associated with heart valve disease. Big mistake. All the cases they reported were phen-fen cases, but they had some cases of heart valve damage with fenfluramine alone, that they failed to mention, and–get this–no cases with phentermine alone. They simply assumed it was the combination of drugs causing the problem, and the *New England Journal of Medicine* let them get away with it. This sloppiness cost Americans billions of dollars in pointless litigation, poisoned the mind of the FDA and deprives Americans to this day of the effective diet medicines they need. The mix-up has never been fixed because the people in authority and journalists in particular have a religious opposition to pills for fat people. They see obesity as a moral failing, not as a disease.

The moralists need not have worried. You can't cure obesity with a hunger-reducing pill anyway, because most of the eating obese Americans do has nothing to do with hunger. Fat men eat big meals. They eat the whole plate, and our plates are big! Fat women eat sugary snacks between meals from loneliness, boredom, overwork and frustration. It's a stereotype I know, but a useful one. I have used it appropriately for sixteen years. Some ten thousand people have lost weight in my clinic and kept the weight off. Phen-pro and the Six Lessons are my tools (see below).

That's enough about that. Weren't there some other diet pills kicking about? Yes. There were.

- Phendimetrazine or Bontril. Still used, but some doctors worry the drug might, rarely, cause primary pulmonary hypertension (PPH). Both fenfluramine and phenmetrazine were linked to PPH in the 1996 case control study by Abenheim.[13] The liver converts phen-*dimetrazine* to phenmetrazine, so wouldn't you worry? There's no published evidence either way, but the

Wyeth Company quietly pulled their Plegine brand of phendimetrazine off the market. Bontril soldiers on.

- Sibutramine or Meridia was a drug with the effect of both phentermine and Prozac in a single drug, in theory. In practice it raised blood pressure. (Phentermine does not[14]) So the FDA limited Meridia to only 15 mg a day, a dose at which it had no Prozac effect. As you might expect, it stopped working after six weeks, the same way phentermine monotherapy does. It's all moot now. Sibutramine was removed from the market by the manufacturer after some damaging European reports linked it to heart disease.[15]

- Orlistat a.k.a. Xenical or Alli partially blocks the absorption of fat from the gut. Since the fat that is not absorbed continues on through the gut to the end, orlistat tends to cause oily diarrhea and malabsorption of fat-soluble vitamins such as D and E. Orlistat never causes much weight loss either, since most fat Americans eat cookies, not fat. Alli is still on the market.

- Topirimate or Topamax is the latest diet drug to be singed by the spotlight of public attention. Topamax came onto the market originally to treat seizures, but it was noticed, in studies, that the more obese subjects had weight loss as a side-effect.[16] Some doctors got the idea to use Topamax for weight-loss in fat people without seizures.[17] Then others got the idea to combine Topamax with phentermine. A combination pill, Qsymia, was approved by the FDA June 2012. It doesn't make sense. Phentermine works only on middle-weight people and Topamax only on the very obese. Who benefits from both drugs?[18]

I could talk about hoodia, ephedra, and Contrave, but what's the point? They never made it to market or they're gone. Chromium, gambogia and B-12 don't work either.

There are many fake medicines on the Internet. Don't be taken in.

Finally, I will explain why fenfluramine caused heart valve disease. Fenfluramine is converted to nor-fenfluramine and nor-fenfluramine binds to 5-HT2B receptors, a serotonin receptor on heart valves.[19] All such drugs in the past caused heart valve problems. About a quarter of people have a higher-than-usual concentration of 5-HT2B receptors on their heart valves. When any of those people takes fenfluramine, their heart valves twist and scar.

Phentermine does not bind to the 5-HT2B receptor, so there have been no cases of phentermine-related heart valve disease[20,21,,22] Even though it's all published, not one doctor or pharmacist in 500 knows any of this.

What to do now?

The true situation with phentermine should be taught to medical students so that as the un-teachable old generation of doctors passes away, the new generation of doctors will be familiar with phentermine. Journalists are a problem, too. They won't do the obesity story straight. They focus on pills and groundless fears. They seek controversy, not truth. They trade on fear.

If you are overweight, you should follow the Six Lessons in my book *Life Between Meals*.

1. Eat less food
2. Cut back carbs, especially sugar
3. Drink a lot more water
4. Weigh yourself every day
5. Stop snacking
6. Eat with friends.

Be a social person. True happiness comes from relationships with good people, not from anything you buy.

Don't be stressed. Give up where you can't win, and move on. Life is more than food. It's art and nature and sports and science, too. Get a life between meals.

Meanwhile, while you are learning all of this, you can take phen-pro. It usually helps.

References

1. Anchors M Fluoxetine is a Safer Alternative to fenfluramine in the Medical Treatment of Obesity. *Arch Intern Med* 1997;157:1270.
2. Anchors M *Safer Than Phen-Fen*, 1997, Prima Publishing, Rocklin CA, 240 pages.
3. Padla D Spoke J. Weight loss comparison between a fluoxetine/ phentermine regimen and select common regimens. *Obes Res* 1997;5:P117.
4. Anchors M Phentermine and fluoxetine are a safe substitute for phen-fen in the treatment of obesity. Eighth International Congress on Obesity, Paris, France August 29-Sept. 3, 1998.
5. Anchors M. Update on the phen-pro combination. *The Bariatrician* Fall 2002, page 17-22.
6. Anchors M. *Life Between Meals*. 2005. Anchors Books, Rockville, MD, 206 pages.
7. Anchors M. Phentermine. Still good after 50 years *The Bariatrician,* Winter 2008, page 13-17.
8. Weintraub M. Long-term weight control: the National Heart, Lung and Blood Institute funded multimodal intervention study. *Clin Pharmacol Therap* 1992; 51:581-585.
9. Patent number 5,795,895, date Aug.18, 1998
10. Sarcasm
11. Connolly H Crary J Mcgoon M et al. Valvular heart disease associated with fenfluramine-phentermine. *NEJM* 1997;337:581-88.

12. Griffen L Anchors M Asymptomatic Mitral and Aortic Valve Disease Is Seen in Half of the Patients Taking Phen-Fen. *Arch Intern Med* 1998;158:102.

13. Abenheim L Moride Y Brenot F et al. Appetite-suppressant drugs and the risk of primary pulmonary hypertension. *NEJM* 1996;335:609-616.

14. Langlois KJ, Forbes JA, Bell GW et al. A double-blind clinical evaluation of the safety and efficacy of phentermine hydrochloride (Fastin) in the treatment of exogenous obesity. *Curr Therap Res* 1974;16:289-296.

15. http://voices.washingtonpost.com/check-up/2010/10/weight-loss_drug_withdrawn.html

16. Ben-Menachem E Axelsen M Johanson EH et al. Predictors of weight loss in adults with topirimate for weight loss. *Obes Res* 2003;11:556-562.

17. Bray GA Hollander P Klein S et al. A 6-month randomized, placebo-controlled dose-ranging trial of topirimate for weight los sin obesity. *Obes Res* 2003;11:722-733.

18. http://www.nytimes.com/2010/10/29/health/policy/29drug.html

19. Rothman RB, Bauman MH, Savage JE et al. Evidence for possible involvement of 5-HT2B receptors in the cardiac valvulopathy associated with fenfluramine and other serotonergic medicines. *Circulation* 2000;102:2836-2841.

20. Rothman RB Baumann MH Dersch et al. Amphetamine-type central nervous system stimulants release norephinephrine more potently than they release dopamine and serotonin. *Synapse* 2001;39:32-41.

21. Griffen L Anchors M "The 'Phen-Pro' Diet Drug Combination is not associated with Valvular Heart Disease." *Arch Intern Med* 1998;158:1278.

22. Rader A, Steelman GM, Westman E. Clinical experience using appetite suppressants and SSRIs. *J Okla State Medical Assoc* 2008;101(8).

MYTH #11

Taking multivitamin vitamin-pills is important.

Fact

Not so much, although a Vitamin D supplement may be important in some people and vitamin B-12 in a few.

Why we should have known better

Healthy human beings have lived for thousands of years, and still do in other countries, without taking vitamin pills. There are vitamins in food and–heaven knows–Americans eat a lot of food. As pointed out in the last myth, the average American eats over 2,700 calories a day. Even if some of it is hotdogs and ice-cream, it's not all hotdogs and ice-cream. Vitamin D is made in the skin in response to sunshine; it is not even necessary to get it in food.

How we got confused

By feeling guilty about what we eat. And our general belief in the primacy of technology over Nature . . . as long as the technology doesn't come from the federal government . . . and it's natural and ecological and it's . . . gosh we're so mixed up.

Below are the daily values for nutritional labeling or DVs for the vitamins, from the 17th Edition of *Food Values of Portions Commonly Used* by Bowes & Church. The DVs are higher and more appropriate than the old recommended minimum daily allowance or RDA. No one says "RDA" anymore.

Vitamin A	5,000 IU
Vitamin B1 (thiamine)	1.5 mg
Vitamin B2 (riboflavin)	1.7 mg
Vitamin B6 (pyridoxine)	2.0 mg

Vitamin B12 (cobalamin)	6.0 mcg
Folate	400 mcg
Vitamin C	60 mg
Vitamin D	400 IU
Vitamin E	30 IU

The next job is to find an estimate of how much of what foods the average American eats. You can't find this on the Internet, but Peter Menzel did a useful picture book. In *Hungry Planet,* he went to 30 countries to photograph an average family together with all the food they eat in an average week.[1] His message was that Americans eat a godzilla amount of food compared to other nations.

Peter gave me three choices of a family to study: (1) the health-conscious Cavens of California, (2) the Willy family of North Carolina who have given up on healthy eating, and (3) the Fernandez family of Texas. I chose the Willy family to study because they seemed most likely to eat 2700 calories, each, per day, the national average.

I started calculating the total amount of each vitamin in the food the Willies ate, using Bowes & Church as a guide.[2] Then I remembered I had less than a century to write this book, so I decided, instead, to focus on folate, the vitamin in lowest supply in the typical diet. Folate comes from fresh leafy green vegetables (*folium*, Latin for leaf).

If you leave out the bread the Willies ate, each family member got only 150 mcg of folate per day, from their average of two bananas a day and some spinach or broccoli spread out through the week. They needed 400 mcg each. Bread came to their rescue. In the flatbread wraps, garlic toast, and two pizzas they consumed, there was an additional 400 mcg of folate. The federal government mandates that folate be added to bread, about 50 mcg per slice.

So even with such limited considerations, the Willies still consumed 550 mcg of folate or 37% more than they needed. The situation is even better than that, though, since the DV of 400 mcg per day for folate was formulated to avert neural tube defects in the fetus in pregnant women. Non-pregnant people don't need so much.

If the Willies would only eat a few more leafy green veg-etables, they wouldn't have to depend so much on bread for folate. In Menzel's book, the Willies ate a green vege-table only once or twice a week. Do you eat vegetables so seldom? I doubt it. If you eat more, and you eat some bread, then you don't need to get folate from vitamin pills.

In many cases the vitamins in real food are absorbed better than their pickled cousins in vitamin pills. Just be-cause a drug company puts 400 IU of folate in a pill does not mean you absorb 400 or 200 or even 50 IU from the pill. Such a fact can only be determined by following the ab-sorption of a tiny amount of radioactively labeled folate in the pill, and such studies are rare. There's no incentive for drug companies to fund such studies.

Folate was the vitamin in lowest supply. Americans get *plenty* of B vitamins in meat, Vitamin A in ubiquitous car-rots, C in orange juice, and vitamin E in fish. Granted, many Americans don't eat much fish, but it's unclear why vitamin E is even a vitamin. It was declared a vitamin originally only because in vitamin E-deficient people there was a build up of pigment in the brain found on autopsy, but the pig-ment had no effect on the individual's function in life.[3] I am aware of no clinical diseases from vitamin E deficiency. A prospective study in JAMA this year even showed a 17% increase in prostate cancer in men taking vitamin E supple-ments. (JAMA 2011;306:1549-1556).

I always wondered, didn't you? what happened to vita-mins F-J. The next named vitamin in the series is vitamin K. What happened to vitamins F-J? Are you worried? I bet if I marketed a vitamin F-J supplement, Americans would buy it. I could be rich, rich.

Switching gears. Some people need vitamin B-12 shots because they have a genetic condition, pernicious anemia, preventing the absorption of vitamin B-12 from the gut. They get monthly B-12 shots from the doctor. But vitamin B-12 has long been available in an orally absorbed form that melts in the mouth. That route is not very efficient, but for most people with pernicious anemia, the orally absorbed form is good enough to avert the need for shots. Unfortunately, most physicians don't know about the oral alternative.

Vitamin D

That leaves us to consider vitamin D. I will begin with the conclusion, because the discussion is so complex. *You may well need to take a vitamin D supplement if you get little sunlight on your skin or if you are elderly. Otherwise, you don't need a supplement.*[3]

Now if you want, you may skip to the next chapter. But for the people who really care about vitamin D–and there are a lot them–here is a concerto in D major . . .

When the UV-B rays in sunshine fall on bare skin, some cholesterol in the skin is converted to vitamin D. Yes, cholesterol, the "bad" stuff you worried about; one more reason it is essential for life.

UV-A rays, on the other hand, don't help with vitamin D and cause sunburn. Fortunately, UV-A is only bad outside between 10 AM and 2 PM when the sun is directly over-head. UV-A is blocked by sunglasses and sunscreen lotions.

Most lotions don't block UV-B. UV-B is not as bad as UV-A, but it's not benign either. UV-B is responsible for photo-aging of the skin, and for basal and squamous cell carcinomas. These two common types of skin cancer are seldom fatal because the cancers metastasize late and are usually caught early. The bad actor in skin cancer is melanoma, but melanoma is (A) rare, (B) genetic in origin and (C) triggered by an amount of sunlight so low you'd never avoid it unless you worked 24-7 in a funeral parlor.

UV-A is blocked by melanin, the brown pigment in the skin of tanned people, or in those people who call themselves "black". Melanin does not block UV-B. Tanned people or "black" people can make vitamin-D from sunlight about as well as "white" people.[4] The human species originated in Africa; it would be strange if the species had developed a skin pigment that blocked vitamin D production.

How much sunlight do you need to produce a sufficient amount of vitamin D? Answer: *four* 4 minute exposures *per week* to the sun on 25% of the body (back and chest), the strength of the sun figured as the strength on a summer day in Denmark.[5] Over-exposure does not create excess vitamin D, because after the first few minutes, extra vitamin D starts to be destroyed in the skin. A balance is achieved.

So unless you live at the North Pole, you get enough vitamin D from the sun; you don't need to take a supplement or get vitamin D from food.

Is that true? Well it's almost true. There's more to the story. Raw vitamin D is quickly converted in the liver to 25-hydroxy-vitamin D or vitamin D_2, the storage form of the vitamin that has little hormone-effect. The truly active form of vitamin D is 1,25-dihydroxy-vitamin D or vitamin D_3. It is made from vitamin D_2 in the kidney in response to *parathyroid hormone*, the hormone regulating the blood level of calcium.

Vitamin D_3 is needed for absorbing calcium from food and funneling calcium into bones. The blood level of calcium must be regulated carefully because calcium determines the strength with which the heart muscle contracts.

I don't understand why so many non-endocrinologists measure blood levels of vitamin D_3 in young people with normal kidneys. The only valid reason to do so is to assess the parathyroid axis, and you can do that better by measuring calcium and parathyroid hormone levels directly. The doctors intending to look for vitamin D deficiency should measure vitamin D_2, the more constant "storage" form of vitamin D, which is not dependent on parathyroid hormone. Vitamin D_2 or 25-hydroxy-vitamin D is the form for which the international normal range of 30-40 ng/ml was set up.

But even measuring vitamin D2 is not a sure-fire way to assess vitamin D *function*, because it has recently been discovered that not all vitamin D_3 is made by the kidneys. Brain, prostate, breast, colon, and many white blood cells have receptors for vitamin D_3 and many of these cells can convert vitamin D_2 to D_3 on their own. This vitamin D_3 is made and consumed locally, so does not factor into the blood level. The local action of vitamin D_3 means that vitamin D is involved in the function of many organs, not just in building bones; and the local action of vitamin D is not reflected in the blood level of vitamin D or parathyroid hormone.

There is a boat-load of evidence connecting vitamin D_2 levels with everything from cancer, heart disease, diabetes, and obesity to resistance to infections. Given what I just told you about the local action of vitamin D, any of it might be true. Any of it might be helped by vitamin D_2 supplementation. But there are no positive randomized controlled trials, and I taught you that such trials are the only ones to get your respect.[6] Retrospective studies and epidemiologic evidence may raise questions, but only randomized controlled trials ever answer them.

What to do now?

It doesn't hurt to take a multiple vitamin once a day. It's a just a waste of money, unless you have a specific vitamin deficiency disease or you are elderly–then it might help something. American vitamin-taking is more about feeling good about oneself, than about biology. If you really want to make the world a better place, send your vitamin pills, instead, to Darfur or Somalia where underfed people need them. Better yet, send them real food.

References

1. Menzel P and D'Aluisio F. *Hungry Planet*. Material World Books, Napa CA, 2005.

2. *Bowe's & Church's Food Values of Portions Commonly Used* (17th Edition) by Jean A. T. Pennington. Lippincott William & Williams, 2000.

3. "Report questions need for 2 diet supplements" by Gina Kolta New York Times November 29, 2010

4. Bogh MKB, Schmedes AV, Philipsen PA *el al*. (2010) Vitamin D production after UVB exposure depends on baseline vitamin D and total cholesterol but not on skin pigmentation. *J Invest Dermatol* 130:546-53

5. Bogh MKB Schmedes AV Philipsen PA *et al*. Vitamin D production depends on ultraviolet-B dose but not on dose rate: a randomized controlled trial. *Exper Dermatol* 2011;20;14-18.

6. LaCroix AZ, Kotchen J, Anderson G, Brzyski R et al. Calcium plus vitamin D supplementation and mortality in postmenopausal women: the Women's Health Initiative calcium-vitamin D randomized controlled trial. *J Gerontol A Biol Sci Med Sci* 2009;64:559-67.

MYTH #12

Antioxidants make you live longer

Fact

I wish it was so. But sorry. No.

Why we should have known better

Because people taking antioxidant pills age as fast as everyone else, and die at the same age as everyone else. Not a single published study giving antioxidants to animals ever extended the maximum lifespan, i.e. changed the aging process itself.

How we got confused

The confusion began with the free radical hypothesis for the aging process.[1] Free radicals are reactive species of oxygen, voraciously attacking big molecules such as DNA and proteins. It would be strange indeed if in four billion years of life on earth, living organisms had not developed a defense against these free radicals. Indeed, thermophilic bacteria live in hot sulfur springs which has lots of free radicals, and they do just fine.[2] Cells make chemicals called free radical scavengers that sop up the free radicals.

Free radicals can't be the cause of aging because closely- related species often have very different lifespans. When opossums in Georgia became isolated on new channel islands created by storms, within a few generations the opossums developed a longer lifespan.[3] The difference was genetic because island opossums kept in captivity still lived 50% longer then mainland opossums kept in captivity. You can't tell me the mainland opossums in captivity were exposed to more free radicals than their island cousins in the cage next door. It was a real genetic change in lifespan induced in a few generations, not by resistance to free radicals but from the absence of predators on the new channel islands.

Are short-living frogs living in the same ditch with long-living turtles exposed to more free radicals than the turtles are? No. Why do parrots outlive canaries? Not because of free radicals, surely. I say, Free All Radicals! Power To The People! Uh oh, flashback.

What to do now?

Stop buying, eating and drinking things because they contain antioxidants. If you like red wine, drink red wine in moderation. If you like dark chocolate, eat it in moderation. You don't have to make up a reason for it. But consume those things in moderation, because everything should be done in moderation except telling the truth.

Coffee has five times as much antioxidants as red wine does.[4] You don't see people rushing out to drink coffee because of the antioxidants. That should show you that the whole antioxidant thing is a sales gimmick.

References

1. http://en.wikipedia.org/wiki/Free-radical_theory Notice that Wikipedia calls it the "free radical *theory* of aging", and you know that is inconsistent with the definition of "theory" on page 19.
2. Qi H, Chen H, Ao J et al. Identification of differentially expressed genes in Sulfobacillus sp. TPY grown on either elemental sulphur or Fe(2+). *J Gen Appl Microbiol.* 2010;56:389-97.
3. Austad S. Taming lions, unleashing a career. *Sci Aging Knowledge Environ* 2002;12:vp3
4. Daglia M Racchi M Papetti A et al. In vitro and ex vivo antihydroxyl radical activity of green and roasted coffee. *J Agric Food Chem* 2004;52:1700-4.

MYTH #13

A low calcium diet, or a low oxalate one, prevents kidney stones.

Fact

Lowering calcium or oxalate in the diet takes away most of the good-tasting things you are used to, and does nothing to prevent kidney stones.

Why we should have known better

Because you never saw these tactics work. And because the Saudis who have a low calcium diet have the highest incidence of kidney stones in the world . . . and the Scandanavians who drink a lot of milk have the lowest.[1]

How we got confused

We relied on the reasonableness of the explanation. Doctors knew that in hyperparathyroidism, a disease in which patients have a very high level of calcium in the blood and urine, the patients indeed have frequent kidney stones.

90% of kidney stones, even from normal people without hyperparathyroidism, are composed of calcium oxalate; so if you reduce the calcium or oxalate in the diet, you ought to be able to reduce the number of kidney stones, right?

It could have turned out that way, but it didn't. I warned you, didn't I? Nature is not simple. Contrary to your expectaitons, a low-calcium diet does not reduce the number of kidney stones.[2] No, it's a *high-calcium* diet that decreases the number of stones.[3] Didn't see that one coming, did you?

But here's a kicker. Taking calcium *supplements* (pills), as opposed to getting extra calcium in food, does increase the number of kidney stones.[3] Why would that be? It is because when calcium and oxalate are ingested together, as they are in food, the calcium and oxalate form an insoluble salt, calcium oxalate, in the gut and neither the calcium nor the oxalate gets absorbed.[4] If you take calcium alone as a pill, there is no oxalate to bind the calcium in the gut, so more of it is absorbed.

If you have kidney stones and gone to the doctor, you have seen that the doctor does a test to measure the levels of calcium and oxalate in your blood. Then, if she is an American doctor, she tells you to cut out as much calcium from your diet as possible. A few weeks later when you return to the office, the blood or urine test is repeated, and now blood or urine calcium is lower, but gadzooks! the oxalate is high. Of course. Without calcium to bind the oxalate in the gut, more oxalate is absorbed, so the blood level is higher.

So the doctor now tells you to cut oxalate out of your diet. She already took milk and cheese away from you;

now the witch wants to take away coffee, tea, spinach and chocolate. The whole thing is an artifact of her first incorrect diet advice. I assure you that reducing the oxalate in your diet will have no effect on your kidney stones.

The effective ways to reduce kidney stones through diet and supplements are to take (A) more water[5], (B) more magnesium[6] and (C) more citrate[6] . The water you'll get from the tap, magnesium from a bottle, and citrate from a bottle or from oranges.

The reason so many Saudis, 20-40%, get kidney stones is dehydration. Arabia is a hot dry country. The southern part of the U.S. is the "stone belt" for the same reason. Osama Bin Laden, a Saudi, had kidney stones, not kidney failure as the newspapers reported. When the newspapers reported he had kidney failure in 2002, I knew they were wrong–I knew what he really had.

Even if the calcium and oxalate in your urine are high, you are unlikely to form a kidney stone unless there is a "seed crystal", a tiny starter crystal, to start the ball rolling. Most urologists believe that the seed crystal is a kernel of uric acid. I don't know where they get this idea from; I can't find a reference for it. It's probably in the category of "reasonable ideas". People who excrete lots of uric acid form stones made entirely of uric acid or its salt, sodium urate. Maybe the existence of uric acid stones gave urologists the idea that sodium urate might be the seed crystal for calcium oxalate stones.

The urologist already took away milk, spinach and brown beverages from you. Her next bright idea, when all that has failed, is to take away meat and salt, because she believes that meat-eaters excrete a lot of uric acid–as indeed they do. Uric acid is the breakdown product of DNA; there's a lot of DNA in meat. In one study where meat and salt were restricted, the number of kidney stones of all types was reduced,[7] but it was only 120 patients, RRR=50% P=0.04. Hmm. Could be true.

But not all of the uric acid in urine comes from meat. A lot of it comes from sugar, especially fructose. Vegetarians, the kind who eat cookies instead of broccoli, get kidney stones too. Sugar doesn't have DNA, so it's not immediately obvious why the uric acid would go up, but pour yourself a drink and listen to Robert Lustig explain it. You'll understand eventually. It took me a while. http://www.youtube.com/watch?v=dBnniua6-oM.

Besides uric acid, the other mainstream idea for a seed crystal is the Randall plaques which appear within the membranes in the kidney. When the plaques eventually erupt through the membrane, they expose their calcium phosphate surface leading to stone formation.[8]

Where do Randall plaques come from? Olavi Kajander of Finland thinks he knows.[9] He thinks they are tiny bacteria called nanobacteria. He has pictures of them in kidneys and kidney stones, in fact in all the kidney stones he examined. Nanobacteria, ancient in origin, were only recently discovered. Extremely small, they are the oysters of the bacterial world; they form a calcium phosphate shell. Look at these pictures . . .

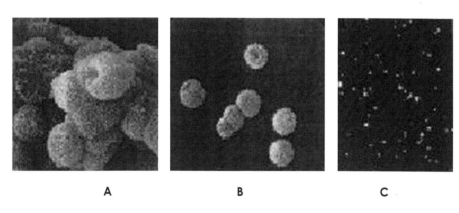

A   B   C

FIG. 12.

A IS AN ELECTRON MICROSCOPE PICTURE OF A KIDNEY STONE. ELECTRON MICROSCOPES ARE VERY POWERFUL AND SHOW VERY TINY STRUCTURES. B IS AN ELECTRON MICROSCOPE PICTURE OF CALCIUM-COATED NANOBACTERIA GROWING IN A CULTURE. SAME MAGNIFICATION. NOTE HOW THEY LOOK LIKE SIMILAR STRUCTURES IN KIDNEY STONES. C IS A PHOTOMICROGRAPH OF THE CUT SURFACE OF A KIDNEY STONES STAINED FOR NANOBACTERIA. THE BACTERIA WERE SEEN IN EVERY STONE.

I hope the world will allow Olavi to establish his hypothesis or rule it out. I myself had calcium oxalate stones every two years from 1972 until 1998 when I read Olavi's article. I put myself on tetracycline 250 mg once a day because I reasoned it might stop the cycle of stone formation by killing nanobacteria and preventing them from getting reestablished. There was no published evidence to guide me on which antibiotic to choose, but tetracycline seemed like a good choice since it was cheap and safe. It has a double negative charge which fits well with the calcium in the shell of the nanobacteria. True, tetracycline is metabolized in the liver and not the kidney, but that did not mean it would be ineffective. Who knew how the nanobacteria got to the kidney? I doubted they ascended from the bladder; other bacteria don't do that. I guessed they came from the blood.

A lot of guessing I know. Quite a departure from my previous insistence on strong evidence, but I am about to make a point. Bear with me.

Anyway I had no stones for ten years, by far the longest stone- free interval of my life. I stopped the tetracycline in 2008 because it had been ten years since I started it and be-cause I knew that stone-formers often stop forming stones when they get really old. I was getting really old.

Mistake! I had two stones in 2010.

During the same period, I prescribed tetracycline to six of my stone-forming patients for whom other prevention strategies had failed. None of them has had another kid-ney stone since then, except one who had stopped taking the medicine.

That's a small "study". You cannot say you are convinced. It's not enough patients. No control group. But remember, I said that scientific evidence consists of two things.

- Well-done scientific experiments
- Extensive long-term practical experience accurately observed by many people

We are now talking about the second box. Extensive experience. Doctors are allowed to think about that. I wish more doctors did, instead of sucking down everything the pharmaceutical companies give them. My clinical experience is a valid form of evidence *for me* to use in conducting my medical practice.

I *should* discuss my discoveries with my local colleagues, which I do, and they should show curiosity, which they often don't . I *should* publish my observations in a journal, but no journal publishes anecdotal findings anymore. The *Archives of Internal Medicine* used to do it–they published my first notice of success with phen-pro–but now the *Archives* rejects such material, because it doesn't come from and isn't screened by the pharmaceutical companies whose advertising pays for the journal.

Once upon a time, doctors subscribed to journals, or their medical libraries did. But now, few journals are funded that way. The journals get their funding now from advertising fees paid by the pharmaceutical companies. Whence comes the money, there goes the loyalty.

What to do now?

If you get kidney stones, I am NOT telling you to take tetracycline. Even I am not sure that trick really works. It is possible that my five patients on tetracycline who never got a stone again, would not have had a stone anyway. It's entirely possible. *It's only five patients.* The subject needs to be properly studied with a randomized controlled trial, which, I am sure no pharmaceutical company will ever do because there's no money in an old, cheap drug like tetracycline.

That is why we need, desperately need for government to fund independent clinical research.

You calcium oxalate stone-formers should drink lots of water, and you should take a potassium-magnesium citrate pill, such as Beelith. Those treatments are proven.

If you are one of the people who form pure uric acid stones, allopurinol may be a good choice for you. It reduces hepatic production of uric acid.

But discuss all of this with your doctor. And do me a favor. Ask them if they have ever heard of Olavi Kajander?

References

1. Romero V Akpinar H Assimos DG. Kidney Stones: A Global Picture of Prevalence, Incidence, and Associated Risk Factors . *Rev Urol* 2010;12:86-96.
2. Trinchieri A Nespoli R Ostini F at al. A study of dietary calcium and other nutrients in idiopathic renal calcium stone formers. *J Urol* 1998;159:654-657.
3. Curhan GC Willett CW, Speizer FE et al. Comparison of dietry calcium with supplemental calcium an other nutrients as factors affecting the risk of kidney stones. *Ann Intern Med* 1997;126:497-504.
4. Liebman M Chai W. Effect of dietary calcium on urinary oxalate excretion after oxalate loads. *Am J Clin Nutr* 1997;65:1453-1459.
5. Borghi L Meschi T Amato F et al. Urinary volume, water and recurrences in idiopathic calcium nephrolithiasis: a 5-year randomized prospective study. *J Urol* 1996;155:839-843.
6. Ettinger B Pak CYC Citron JT. Potassium-magnesium citrate is an effective prophylaxis against recurrent calcium oxalate nephrolithiasis. *J Urol* 1997;158:2069-2073.
7. Borghi L Shianchi T Meschi T et al. Comparison of two diets for the prevention of recurrent stones in idiopathic hypercalciuria. *N Engl J Med* 2002;346:77-84.
8. Evan AP Coe FL Lingeman JE et al. Mechanism of formation of human calcium oxalate renal stones on Randall's plaque. *Anat Rec (Hoboken)*. 2007;290:1315-1323.
9. Kajander O Ciftcioglu N Miller-Hjelle MA et al. Nanobacteria: controversial pathogens in

nephrolithiasis and polycystic kidney disease. *Current Opinion in Nephrology and Hypertension* 2001;10:445-452.

MYTH #14

Biphosphonates, such as Fosamax, Actonel, Boniva and others, treat osteoporosis by reversing it. Many, even most, older women should take a bisphosphonate to arrest and reverse osteoporosis.

Fact

Bisphosphonates are bone hardeners, not bone-builders. Taken too long, they make the long bones brittle and fragile.[1]

Why we should have known better
Bisphosphonates reduce spinal compression fractures where the line of force is along the line of the bone (vertebra) itself, and prevent some hip fractures, but bisphosphonates do not prevent fractures in limbs when lateral forces are involved. They may even increase fractures there, and the fractures heal poorly. The bones fracture in a characteristic spiral pattern, for the good reason that they can't compress—they can only splinter.[2-6] Most of the references cited here are from foreign journals, a case study in how difficult it has become to get adverse information about American drugs into American journals.

How we got confused
By allowing long term treatment (>5 years) of a large number of people to proceed on the basis of short-term (<2 year) studies. Long-term studies are expensive, and pharmaceutical companies are locked in a race to

get their product out first. They put pressure on the FDA to approve their drug. The FDA is under pressure to help sick people and prevent injuries. So the FDA approves medicines for a large number of people based on studies of a few–only a thousand were studied before Mevacor was approved–and the FDA allows long duration of use on the basis of short-term studies. Actually what the FDA says is this:

The FDA has recognized that the FD&C Act does not limit the manner in which a physician may use an approved drug. Once a product has been approved for any marketing, a physician may choose to prescribe it for uses or in treatment regimens or patient populations that are not included in approved labeling. The FDA also observes that accepted medical practice includes drug use that is not reflected in approved drug labeling.

The American people become the testing ground for new drugs and new uses of drugs. I have no objection to this idea in principle; given the constraints of time and money, there is no other good way to approve drugs. But for the system to work in practice, there must be an *honest* system in place to watch for adverse effects of new drugs after the drugs are released, and THAT we do not have.

Take the case of my friend Wilhelmina, 62 years old, standing on a stool, leaning over to get something from the top of her refrigerator, putting lateral stress on her right leg. All of us do something like this every day. It wasn't much stress–Wilhelmina is a tiny, lean, long-distance runner. I could pick her up with a feather. Poor Wilhelmina. Her femur, the thickest bone in her body, splintered in mid-shaft. Such things do not occur naturally.

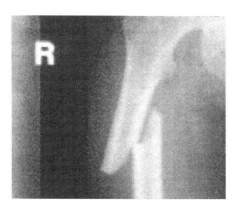

FIGURE 13.

CLASSIC SPIRAL FEMORAL FRACTURE OF BISPHOSPHONATE OVERUSE.

Notice that the bone in the picture looks dense; the cortex, the outer layer of bone, is white in color, not the ghost grey of osteoporosis. The grey part seen in the middle of the bone in the picture is the bone marrow. It's the white outer layer, cortex, that gives bone its strength. The reason Wilhelmina's bone looked white in the x-ray, instead of the gray it was before, was that she had been taking bisphosphonates.

On a routine bone scan years before, Wilhelmina had been found to have osteoporosis; her doctor, following usual procedure, had prescribed a bisphosphonate for her. Doing so he reduced the chance of spinal compression fractures, in which the vertebrae squash down like biscuits under a fist. Spinal compression fractures give us so many short, bent-over old people. Accidents, Pagets disease and ankylosing spondylitis contribute their share, too, but spinal compression fractures are the main culprit.

The doctor reduced the chance of a hip fracture, too; they are always in the top five causes of disability and death in old people. Overall, the doctor did Wilhelmina a favor by prescribing the bisphosphonate . . . for the first year . . . and the second. By that time, her T Score on the duplex scan, which measures the amount of calcium in the bone, had returned to normal limits.

Let me explain why. To the naked eye bone looks like permanent solid stuff, like granite. But the microscope structure looks like a sponge, lots of little fibers criss-crossing. The fibers are called *trabeculae*. The trabeculae are strong, because they are full of calcium. Protein is there to hold the calcium in place.

Over time, with repeated stresses from normal daily living, more and more of the trabeculae fracture, i.e. the bone develops tiny microcracks. Nature has an answer for this; bone is normally, continually turning over. Little cells called *osteoclasts* eat up the old bone. Other cells called *osteoblasts* follow behind, filling in the space with new trabeculae. Over time the trabeculae acquire calcium and harden.

In smokers, and in non-smokers genetically destined to develop osteoporosis, there is overactivity of the osteoclasts. Slowly over time the bone contains fewer and fewer trabeculae.

Bisphosphonates inhibit the action of the osteoclasts. That's why doctors hoped the drug would restore the balance. Unfortunately the action of osteoblasts is tightly linked to that of osteoblasts. Slow down one, and you slow down the other.

Over time, as people take biphosphonates their T score, the measure of bone mineralization (calcification) measured with the duplex scan, increases, and their risk of spine and hip fractures goes down for two reasons.

- The trabeculae of bisphosphonate-takers are frozen in time, while the untreated people continue the normal process of breaking down bone (osteoclasts) without adequate replacement of bone (osteoblasts), the same process that caused osteoporosis in the first place. The T score is based on the average bone density for the patient's age-group. So if

the treated people stay the same and the untreated people go down, the T score goes up, *not* because the treated people got any better but because the untreated people got worse.
- In the first year or two of bisphosphonate, mineralization does increase in absolute terms as new bone that was laid down, before the bisphosphonate stopped everything, becomes calcified.

For all these reasons the risk of fracture goes down in the first few years of bisphosphonate use. But notice, the normal process of replacing trabeculae-with-microcracks with new, uncracked bone stops. Over time, more and more of the trabeculae in the bone contain tiny cracks. Eventually the whole structure can give way and a fracture occurs.

What to do now?

Patients should be put on bisphosphonates only if they have established osteoporosis, placing them at real risk for spinal compression fractures and hip fractures. They should take the bisphosphonate for only two years, unless there is an extremely good reason to continue longer. They will benefit by hardening their bone in the first two years, benefit that is long-lasting. And not enough time to acquire too many microcracks. But continuation beyond that point risks fractures other than hip and spine.

As always, the information I give you is not meant to supplant the advice of your personal physician. But if your doctor disagrees with me, ask him or her if they have ever heard of Susan Ott.

References

1. Ott S. New treatments for brittle bones. *Ann Intern Med* 2004;141:406-7.

2. Ali T Jay RH. Spontaneous femoral shaft fracture after long-term alendronate. *Age Ageing* 2009;38:625-6.

3. Bamrungsong T Pongchaiyakul C J Bilateral atypical femoral fractures after long-term alendronate therapy: a case report. Med Assoc Thai. 2010;93:620-4.

4. Capeci CM Tejwani NC. Bilateral low-energy simultaneous or sequential femoral fractures in patients on long-term alendronate therapy. *J Bone Joint Surg Am*. 2009;91:2556-61.

5. Goddard MS, Reid KR Johnston JC *et al*. Atraumatic bilateral femur fracture in long-term bisphosphonate use. *Orthopedics* 2009 Aug;32(8). pii: orthosupersite.com/view.asp?rID=41933.   doi: 10.3928/01477447-20090624-27.

MYTH #15

Taking addictive drugs turns people into addicts.

Fact

Addicts are born, not made. The propensity to abuse drugs is genetic and cultural. The factors are already in place before a drug is ever taken. The reason this is important is that doctors are terribly, terribly frightened of giving adequate pain-relieving medicines to patients in severe pain or anxiety-reducing medicines to people with severe anxiety, out of an unreasonable fear of making the patient an addict.

Even state medical boards are ahead of the doctors on this one. They are begging doctors to give adequate pain relief to patients in pain. Doctors are sued for not giving enough pain medicine. Inadequate pain relief is an important cause of increased morbidity and mortality.

Not giving adequate pain relief is a violation of the Hippocratic oath. Why do so many doctors persist in such dereliction of duty? The causes are rooted in fear, inadequate study and in some doctors, false religion.

Why we should have known better

Many of us have had a broken bone, gallstone, kidney stone, migraine or other cause of severe pain and felt relieved when the doctor finally prescribed Percocet or gave a Demerol shot. We did not thereafter buy a hookah and look for our next "hit" of drug. We did not lie about our drug use or alter prescriptions. We did not. But we assume other people do.

But the majority of people are normal–that's what "normal" means. Normal people do not get addicted after a few experiences with opiate pain relievers or with Xanax for a panic attack. Let's define a few terms here.

"Narcotic" A vague, obsolete term never used by actual doctors now

"Opiate" Any medicine derived from the opium poppy. Examples: morphine, codeine, oxycodeine. The term is loosely used to describe medicines such as Demerol that are completely artificial.

"Drug tolerance" The tendency of some drugs to have reduced effectiveness over time.

"Pseudotolerance" The false-appearance of tolerance occurring not because the drug is becoming less effective, but because the physical disease being treated is getting worse.

"Drug withdrawal" The temporary, unpleasant side-effects that occur when some drugs are discontinued. The symptoms can be serious or not serious.

"Drug dependency" Being at a point in the course of treatment when stopping the drug will cause withdrawal symptoms.

"Drug addiction" Abusing drugs in the sense of taking them without the doctor's consent or in ways the doctor would not approve. Such patients often raise the dose on their own, or go to other doctors to get more medicine without telling either doctor about the other. Addicts forge prescriptions, lie, cheat or steal. Most addicts show true drug tolerance and dependency as well, but the key points of the definition are . . .

- continued use of a drug in the face of known or knowable adverse consequences
- anti-social behaviors

The definition from the American Society of Addiction Medicine is as follows . . .

Addiction is a primary, chronic disease of brain reward, motivation, memory and related circuitry. Dysfunction in these circuits leads to characteristic biological, psychological, social and spiritual manifestations. This is reflected in the individual pursuing reward and/or relief by substance use and other behaviors. *The addiction is characterized by impairment in behavioral control, craving, inability to consistently abstain, and diminished recognition of significant problems with one's behaviors and interpersonal relationships.* [Italics added]. Like other chronic diseases, addiction can involve cycles of relapse and remission. Without treatment or engagement in recovery activities, addiction is progressive and can result in disability or premature death.

Most of you reading this book do not have this largely genetic disease--the tendency to drug abuse.

What to do now?
Doctors should not deny adequate pain-relieving or anxiety-reducing medicines to patients with pain or anxiety. The use of such medicines should, nevertheless, be monitored and carefully documented. Patients should be *appropriately* warned about addiction. Medicines should be cut off or an appropriate referral made at the first sign of addiction or illegal diversion of medications.

But there is no reason to frown or make patients feel like criminals for their *appropriate* drug use. Doctors, read your

Hippocratic Oath. Treat the patient or refer them to someone else who will.

MYTH #16

Stepping on a rusty nail causes tetanus, so tetanus must
have something to do with metal, right?

Fact

Tetanus has nothing to do with metal.

Why we should have known better

Stepping on a rusty nail can cause tetanus, yes, but any
deep, dirty wound can. Tetanus is rare since the vaccine
is so effective. Only 90 cases per year in the whole U.S.
each year. Most cases occur in unvaccinated children and
elderly burn victims.

How we got confused

When I was practicing family practice, fairly often I got
people in the office who had grazed themselves with a clean
knife or stuck themselves with a pin. They were panicked
that they were going to get tetanus from the metal, and
begged me for a tetanus shot. I tried to calm them down.

Where does this paranoia come from? There must have
been someone in the past, probably named Willy, who
stepped on a nail and got "lockjaw". Willy was an important man in the community, too, because people never
forgot the experience.

People! Tetanus has nothing to do with metal! Tetanus
occurs when a small number of anaerobic bacteria, called
Clostridium tetani, grow in a deep wound, not open to the

air, or in a burn area with lots of devitalized tissue. Oxygen kills *C. tetani.*

The bacteria itself is not a problem, but the bug releases a toxic protein, called tetanus toxin, that attaches to muscle fibers and forces them into sustained contraction. Hence the old term "lockjaw".

When your doctor gives you a tetanus shot, they are injecting an inactive form of the toxin, called toxoid. The body forms antibodies to the toxoid, so that in the future if *C. tetani* is growing in a wound, the toxin formed is snapped up by the antibody before the toxin has time to reach the muscle cells.

Obviously you have to have enough antibody in your blood at the time to sop up all the toxin. It's not a case where you can wait for the body to build up immunity. That's why a tetanus shot at the time of the injury doesn't do much good. The tetanus shot given to you by the doctor at the ER after a dog bite is useless. It hurts and costs you money. If the doctor really wants to boost your immediate supply of antibodies, she should give you an infusion of blood plasma. I doubt that is ever done since the risk of the transfusion exceeds the risk of getting tetanus. There's only 90 cases of tetanus in 300,000,000 Americans each year.

The reason elderly victims sometimes get tetanus is because by their advanced age, their supply of anti-tetanus toxin antibodies has diminished. The CDC was considering dropping the recommendation to get a tetanus booster every ten years throughout life, in part because people weren't complying with the recommendation anyway, and in part because even in the absence of regular boosters, young and middle-aged adults so seldom get tetanus.

The CDC discussed giving up on the regular boosters in young people, relying on the immunity gained from their childhood shots to protect them, in exchange for insisting on a single tetanus booster at age 60. I wonder what ever happened to that debate? They never reported anything out.

What to do now?

If tetanus boosters don't bother you, you should get some boosters as an adult, particular around age 60. If they bother you a lot, forget about them.

Don't panic every time you get nicked by a clean piece of metal. If the doctor in the ER gives you a tetanus shot after the family dog nips your leg, well, you probably needed the tetanus booster anyway. But if you know that you are allergic to tetanus toxoid or get bad reactions from the shots, don't let the ER doc give you a tetanus booster after a dog bite. Cleaning and opening the wound to air, topical antiseptics and sometimes antibiotics are the best way to avoid the risk of tetanus.

References

1. http://www.cdc.gov/mmwr/preview/mmwrht-ml/00022879.htm

MYTH #17

Regular mammograms reduce deaths from breast cancer by picking up the cancer early when it can be effectively treated.

Fact

Not so. Sorry.

Why we should have known better

The survival of breast cancer victims who got mammograms or those who didn't is still the same, despite widespread compliance with the national recommendations for getting mammograms. Nevertheless, you will see below that mammograms may have reduced the actual incidence of breast cancer through a mechanism you'd never expect.

How we got confused

It seems so reasonable that if we could see breast cancer in an early stage while it is still small, and cut the cancer out, the cancer would be cured. The image is so seductive that it is hard to give up. But give it up we must.

In the Health Insurance Plan trial in New York City in the seventies and early eighties, 62,000 women aged 40-70 were randomly divided into two groups. Half of the women were *offered* annual mammograms and physical examination. The majority of the women offered the screening took it. The other half of the women were simply observed, which meant, in practice, that no one did anything unless the patient complained of something. Over ten years of the study, 299 breast cancers were found. Only 132 of them were detected by mammography alone. For the other 167, physical exam alone would have been sufficient.

The number of women dying from breast cancer in the mammography group was 93. The number in the observation-only group was 133. All-cause deaths were not reported. From the data that was reported you can see that there was a relative risk reduction of 133-93/133 = 30%.

But what was the absolute risk reduction? The closest we can come is to say that after 10 years, 99.7% of the mammography group did not die from breast cancer, and 99.6% of the control group did not die from breast cancer. That's only a 0.1% difference. And remember the women at the start of the study were only *offered* mammography, not required to do it. Not all of the women agreed. What if those with a family history of breast cancer were more likely to agree to mammography? Then even the 0.1% difference in survival may not have been real.

And that's the biggest study we have! Sorry it's so old. You can't find new studies on this issue because doctors have been so convinced mammography is good that they have been unwilling to do a real control group. Even if the doctors were willing, the general public would not be willing. They have been so brainwashed about the benefit of mammograms that no women would consent to be in a control group.

In Europe the public is not so zealously pro-technology; it is still possible to do real studies on mammography there.[2] A recent study in Denmark showed that mammography was ineffective.[3] The news was big news in the media for a short time in 2010. Have you forgotten all the hoopla? See how life settles back into the sleepy rhythm of following doctor's advice, and doctors following the radiologist's advice or that of the pharm company. No one reading or thinking. No ripple of dissent. Science, real science, seems so pointless to me sometimes. Little has changed since the days of Dr. *Arrowsmith* in Sinclair Lewis' novel. Or since Aristotle.

But don't get depressed! A few pages down I will give you happy news–the incidence of breast cancer in the U.S. and Europe did, in fact, go down between 1990 and 2000, and it was probably because of mammograms. You will be surprised by the reason.

But before we get there, I want to show you more about mammograms. If you screen 1000 women between the ages of 40 and 50, this is what you get . . .

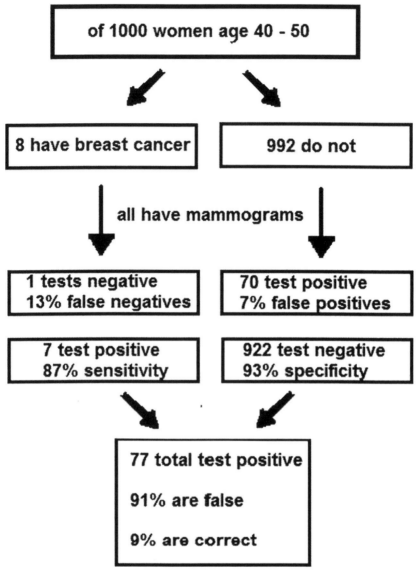

FIGURE 14.

MAMMOGRAM ACCURACY EXPOSED AND CLARIFIED

I need to define sensitivity and specificity. **Sensitivity** shows how good a test is at finding the disease. **Specificity** shows how sure we are that a positive test really means the disease is there.

sensitivity = (true positives)/(false negatives + true positives)
specificity = (true negatives)/(false positives + true negatives)

Let us remind ourselves that the current recommendation from the National Cancer Institute and the American Cancer Society is to get annual mammograms after age 40.

Now look at the chart. In this group of 1000 young women getting mammograms, 77 of them will be told they have a positive or abnormal mammogram. They will be scared. They will go on to a needle biopsy or open surgical biopsy requiring anesthesia. Let's say the rest of the treatment-system works perfectly, and we save all 7 of the true positives. That means saving 0.7% of the total group screened.

But what of the other 70 people? The quality of their life has been permanently altered by the brush with cancer. They still won't be sure they don't have the disease. They will go for more and more tests for breast cancer and for other things. Some become medical invalids.

Stress and uncertainty itself lower resistance to diseases of all types. How many of the 70 false positive women will be affected, severely or fatally? This might be a good time to re-read the wonderful Foreword to this book by Malcolm Kendrick.

But we know that early detection means little for cure. Joel Kauffman writes:

"The authors, Skrabanek and McCormick [reference #2 in this chapter] think that the theory behind breast cancer screening is flawed because a tumor that can be felt (become palpable) has been growing for a mean time of 8 years. Early detection by mammography by two years at most can only be valuable if metastasis is confined to years 6 through 8. There is no reason to think this is the case."

And John Lee MD in his book wrote:

"For a breast cancer tumor to become large enough to be detected by palpation, the cancer has usually been growing for about ten years. If found one year earlier by mammography, the cancer has been growing for about nine years, which is plenty of time to spawn metastases if the cancer is prone to do that."

You must understand that cancer does not grow linearly; it grows geometrically, i.e. 1 cell, 2 cells, 4 cells, 8 cells, etc.

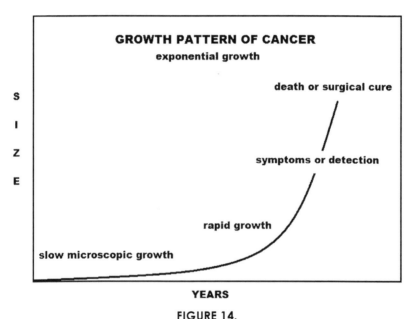

FIGURE 14.

GRAPH SHOWING THE STAGES OF GEOMETRIC GROWTH OF A TUMOR

Cancers remain microscopic in size for a long time before starting to enlarge rapidly. That's how they remain undetected for so long before being found by palpation or mammography. All while they remain small, they can be spreading metastases.

But good news! The incidence of breast cancer death has actually declined! In 1935, the annual incidence was 26.2 out of 100,000 women in the U.S., in 1992 after adjusting for longer lifespan the incidence was the same 26.2 per 100,000. *But in 2000 the incidence was just 18.3 per 100,000.*

Why the drop? The treatment hadn't gotten better. As noted in chapter 2, surgery and chemotherapy have only improved the five-year survival, not the ten-year survival or the fifteen. In any case, better treatment would change the prevalence of breast cancer, not the incidence. The *incidence* itself has gone down. Fewer people get breast cancer at all, not just fewer dying from it.

Dr. Kauffman and others believe the cause of the reduction in incidence of breast cancer is the mere fact of the exposure to x-rays in mammograms and diagnostic chest x-rays, a process called hormesis. **Hormesis** occurs when low-dose radiation induces cells to make more of the enzymes needed to repair damaged DNA. This would do little to cure a cancer already in progress, but would do a lot to keep cancer from getting started.

The existence of hormesis is not universally accepted, I must tell you, but there is good evidence for it. We did not see the reduction in incidence in breast cancer until about ten years after mammograms became widely accepted in the U.S. That makes sense since it takes ten years for breast cancer to grow from a single bad cell to a mass detectable by palpation or mammogram.

Further evidence for the hormesis explanation is that the reduction in breast cancer incidence has not persisted. It went back up in the 2000-2010 period, because in the nineties, we reduced the strength of the x-rays in mammograms, unwittingly reducing the hormetic effect, allowing more cancers to develop in the 2000-2010 period.

So we arrive at the weird conclusion that we can reduce breast cancer deaths best by doing mammograms, exposing the breast to low-dose radiation, but *not* looking at the film to see the results. Ha, and you were going to say that Nature is simple! Nature is not simple.

What to do now?

I am not proposing to expose breasts to x-rays for the hormetic effect without a lot more well-done scientific studies. Even if it was determined it was the best thing to do, you would have an impossible task convincing American women to irradiate their breasts.

The women already worry about the sanity of doctors given their recent flip-flops on many issues. If we told women to irradiate their breasts to prevent cancer, I think they would stop listening to us altogether.

Doing mammograms and so many biopsies is not a good idea until we have better treatments for breast cancer. I don't see the value of mutilating so many healthy women physically and psychologically to garner a few more months or weeks for a few breast cancer victims. Once again, read the Foreword to this book.

References

1. Robin ED. *Matters of Life and Death: Risks and Benefits of Medical Care*. 1984. Stanford, CA Alumni Association
2. Skrabanek P McCormick J. *Follies and Fallacies in Medicine*. Tarragon Press, Glasgow, Scotland 1989
3. Jøørgensen KJ, Zahl PH, Gøøtzsche PC. Breast cancer mortality in organised mammography screening in Denmark: comparative study. *BMJ* 2010;340:1241.

MYTH #18

Balloon angioplasties and the insertion of stents into coronary arteries prevent heart attacks and save lives.

Fact

Hardly at all, and coronary artery bypass grafts don't work either, except, a little, in a small subgroup with "left main disease" (I will explain all of this). Former President Bill Clinton is alive in spite of his coronary artery bypass graft (CABG), not because of it.

How I learned better

On July 24, 2004 a sunny Saturday morning, I was sitting in the National Library of Medicine in Bethesda, Maryland, leisurely putting in the last references in the manuscript of my book *Life Between Meals* when I felt the urge to go to the bathroom. About ten minutes after that I began to have chest and neck pain and feel woozy. I knew I was having a heart attack. I looked at my watch–it was 10:15 AM. I estimated that the first symptoms had occurred around 10:05. I told the librarian I was having a heart attack, dial 911 and guard my laptop. Then I passed out.

The next thing I remember was the EMTs arriving at 10:30 AM. The EMTs transported me to Suburban Hospital, the excellent hospital next door to the National Library of Medicine. To make a short story even shorter, by 11 AM, the cardiologist had performed a balloon angioplasty on me and installed a stent to keep the artery open. The procedure was performed within the "golden hour" as they say.

To be continued . . .

* * *

I have to explain. In a balloon angioplasty the doctor threads a tiny catheter (tube) into the blood clot blocking an artery–into the clot itself–then inflates the balloon at the end of the catheter to squash the clot against the artery wall. A small metal mesh tube, called a stent, is now usually left in place to keep the artery open.

I always thought the idea of keeping arteries open with a wire cage was a little wooly, because what would keep a new clot from forming at the site almost immediately? The balloon angioplasty without the stent did not work–I knew that–the artery just plugged up again right away.[1]

When doctors replace a sick cardiac valve with a mechanical valve, the patients are always put on Coumadin, a major blood thinner, the rest of their life to keep clots from forming on the device. Why wouldn't the metal stent cause the formation of blood clots, too? Doctors explain that in a few weeks or months the body deposits a layer of new cells over the stent, i.e. the stent becomes epithelialized, so that a smooth surface of cells faces the bloodstream and not the bare metal.

I point out that the body also deposited a layer of cells over the flattened clot material in the old stent-less procedure, too, but that did not make that procedure really work.[1] Besides, what's to keep a clot from forming on the stent right away before the stent gets epithelialized?

The answer is . . . nothing. So doctors and companies spent a lot of time developing stents coated with drugs to inhibit clotting. These are called "drug-eluting stents".

The drug-eluting stents were a boondoggle initially because the drug on the stents kept the stents from being epithelialized. People with the coated stents had to take Plavix and aspirin, "blood thinners" actually platelet inhibitors, much longer. Doctors continued to tinker with drug-eluting stents until finally–they say–they got it right. Maybe they have. I haven't been following the subject closely. I've lost interest. As my story continues, you will see why . . .

* * *

My story continues. A few months later, I had an exercise nuclear stress test. They injected me with a tiny amount of a nuclear isotope and set me to exercise on a treadmill. While I was huffing and puffing away, they took a movie of the radioactively-labeled blood coursing through my heart.

I looked at the film with my cardiologist. He seemed pleased with the results, but I asked . . .

Dr. Anchors. What's that big dark spot on the back of my heart?

Dr. Willy (not his real name): Oh, that's the scar.

Dr. Anchors. What scar!

Dr. Willy. You have a scar on your heart, from the heart attack.

Dr. Anchors. Why do I have such a big scar? I got to the hospital right away. All the conditions were ideal.

Dr. Willy. There's usually some scar.

Dr. Anchors. But that's a big scar. I thought the purpose of the angioplasty was to prevent loss of heart muscle.

Dr. Willy. It is.

Dr. Anchors. But it didn't work.

Dr. Willy. It doesn't always work.

Dr. Anchors. Does it ever work?

I saw on the video that the back of my heart was not contracting the way healthy muscle does. I don't think I got any benefit from the angioplasty.

And you know. Let's think about it. No one rushes to put a stent into a patient having a stroke. Because we all know that ten minutes after a stroke begins, the brain tissue downstream from the clot is dead. Restoring the blood flow forty minutes later won't bring the dead tissue back to life.

Why is it not the same with heart muscle tissue? It is. Sort of. The heart muscle is more resilient than brain tissue–it can tolerate low oxygen conditions longer–but not so much longer that the heart muscle can withstand anoxia for an hour. In fact no study has shown that angioplasty has saved a life. I will support my claim with data.

* * *

Before I get to that however, let me comment on an older procedure, the coronary artery bypass surgery (CABG), the procedure Bill Clinton had. The CABG is useless in the setting of a person actively having a heart attack. It is used in people with partially blocked arteries in danger of having a heart attack in the future. Basically, doctors borrow a short stretch of vein or artery from elsewhere in the body and sew it in to provide a bypass route around the narrowed patches of coronary artery.

The CASS Registry was a long-term follow-up study of patients with serious coronary artery disease.[2] Fifteen years into the study the results were as follows:

12,4562 men and 2,366 women studied.

75% of the men ended up having CABG, 72% of the women.

The survival rate for the men with CABG was 52%.

The survival rate for the men on medical therapy alone was 50%.

This means that among men who had a bypass, 2.0% fewer men were dead after 15 years. But the death rate from surgery was 2.5%. Therefore after 15 years, no men's lives had been saved.

The survival rate for the women with CABG was 48%.

The survival rate for women with medical therapy alone was 50%.

This means that among women who had a bypass, 2.0% more were dead after 15 years. The death rate from surgery was 5.3% for women. That means 7.3% *more* women were dead if they had bypass.

While the CASS study did not dampen the enthusiasm of most rank-and-file cardiac surgeons, who were making so much money, darlings of the media, the results did bother the conscience of some surgeons. They searched for a subgroup of patients for whom bypass would provide real benefit.

They found one–the group with blockage in the left main artery, the big pipe running down the front of the heart feeding blood to the left ventricle, the chamber of the heart that pumps blood directly to the body. 85% of that group survived five years after the surgery, compared to only 65% of the group treated medically without the surgery.[3] (Yes, back in the early eighties, they still did real control groups.) Surgery's 85% is not quite as impressive as it looks–and mind you, it doesn't look so impressive–because patients dying in surgery were not counted. The number dying in surgery varied from 2-10% in various series. The honest thing would have been to deduct that number from surgery's 85% survival, and then you'd get, what?

And that was their "best" group!

I want to observe that both the 85% and 65% five-year survival rates were pretty poor. The patients getting bypass back in the eighties were some pretty sick puppies. You can understand the surgeon's desperation to help them.

Recently surgeons, with some massaging of the data, have identified a second group of patients for bypass surgery, i.e. those with triple-vessel or multiple vessel disease. The amount of improvement there wasn't as "good" as with left main disease, but was still statistically significant, though it's hard to say–the surgeons by then had stopped doing any control groups since it was considered unethical not to do some procedure. The survival rates in the surgical series were better, since they were doing bypass surgery on people not as ill to begin with. the survival would have been better in the control groups, too, if they had done any.

* * *

Balloon angioplasty has largely replaced bypass surgery because (1) it is safer and faster. (2) It can be done in the setting of an acute heart attack. And (3) the interventional cardiologist can do the procedure without the aid of a surgeon if all goes well, which it usually does. With so much experience, balloon angioplasty has become a relatively safe procedure.

My quibble is not with the safety of balloon angioplasty, but with its necessity. The trouble is that when patients survive after angioplasty, they are counted as a success for the procedure. When patients without angioplasty die, that too is considered an argument for angioplasty. Angioplasty always gets the credit and never the blame. It's not fair. That's why I wish the doctor-scientists in this area still did double-blind control groups. They consider the basic argument, stent or no stent, settled. They are only looking for the best way to go about it. But the argument is not settled! They just stopped looking.

Look at Kadel et al. 1993 [4]. This German paper is often cited as evidence for the success of angioplasty. 798 patients with single vessel disease who had angioplasty were evaluated up to 8 years after their procedure. The immediate success rate, i.e. the number showing restored blood flow to the previously blocked area, was 81%. That means 19% of the time the balloon didn't unblock the artery to begin with. Keep that group in mind as we go on; it will serve as a control. The frequency of severe complications during the procedure was 7%. Two patients died (0.3%).

The 8-year survival of the patients with successful angioplasty was 97.2%. The survival of the patients whose arteries were not reopened with angioplasty was 88.9%. The difference is significant at only the .04 level. I warned you about "iffy" p values. There is one chance in 25 that this result could have occurred from chance alone. Moreover, think about it, the group in whom the angioplasty was unsuccessful at restoring flow may have been sicker than the group with flow-restored. So naturally their survival might have been 8.5% worse (97.2-88.9/97.2=8.5%).

To me the impressive thing is that 88.9% of the patients who had no restoration of flow survived! It seems the artery-blockage they had was not so dangerous after all.

And the patients with unsuccessful angioplasty underwent the same surgical risks as the patients with successful angioplasty. So without the procedure 89.5% of them would have survived (89.2 + 0.3); or possibly even more since it is known that the mere fact of getting angioplasty weakens the coronary vasculature. Patients post-angioplasty have substantially higher mortality in any subsequent surgery.[5]

Kadel did show that the patients with successful angioplasty had fewer symptoms subsequently–less chest pain and fatigue–than those with failed angioplasty (86.8% vs. 59.5% p<.0001). And more people with successful angioplasty were still working (75.4% vs. 56.9% p<.001) after 8 years. But none of that impresses me because it is likely that the patients who could not complete angioplasty originally were sicker to begin with.

There is no substitute for doing a real, randomized control group!

The Kadel study did not use stents, but it was the most recent study I could find that had anything like a real control group. You can think though, that it would have made no difference if stents had been used. Al Suwaidi et al showed us that . . .

The 23 trials in Al Suwaidi et al. enrolled 10,347 patients, with 5130 patients randomized to receive stent and 5217 patients randomized to receive balloon angioplasty . . . *No significant difference* was observed between the stent group and PTCA [angiography without stent] group in the rates of death or myocardial infarction.[6]

What to do now?

No funding agency should ever sponsor a clinical trial without a proper control group unless there is an adequate reason why a control can't be done.

I am not going to tell you what you should do about your heart because I am not your doctor. But I will tell you what I will do. I will not have another balloon angioplasty, and I will never submit to a bypass.

References

1. Foley DP Hermans WM Rensing BJ et al. Restenosis after percutaneous transluminal coronary angioplasty. *Herz* 1992;17:1-17.
2. Davis K Chaitman B Ryan T et al. Comparison of 15 year survival for men and women after initial medical or surgical treatment of coronary artery disease: a CASS registry study. *J Am Coll Cardiol* 1995;25:1000-1009.
3. Hadler NM. *Worried Sick: A Prescription for Health in an Overtreated America.* University of North Carolina Press, 2008.
4. Kadel C Vallbracht C Buss F et al. Long-term follow-up after percutaneous transluminal coronary angioplasty in patients with single-vessel disease. *Am Heart J* 1992;124:1159-1169.

5. Bonaros N, Hennerbichler D, Friedrich G et al. Increased mortality and perioperative complications in patients with previous elective percutaneous coronary interventions undergoing coronary artery bypass surgery. *Thorac Cardiovasc Surg* 2009;137:846-852.

6. Al Suwaidi J Holmes DR Jr Salam AM et al. Impact of coronary artery stents on mortality and nonfatal myocardial infarction: meta-analysis of randomized trials comparing a strategy of routine stenting with that of balloon angioplasty. *Am Heart J* 2004;147:815-822.

MYTHS NOT GIVEN A FULL SECTION

Myth. Childhood vaccines cause **autism**.

Fact. Not so.

Proof. From a test on the amniotic fluid, we can tell that a fetus has the gene(s) for autism, more than a year before the resulting child receives any vaccine.

Reference. http://www.research-horizons.cam.ac.uk/ spotlight/amniocentesis--a-key-to-identify-autism-in-the-womb-.aspx

* * *

Myth. Childhood vaccines cause **ADD**, or sugar does, or something does. ADD can't just be natural.

Fact. Why can't it be natural?

Proof. The fetus that will become a child with ADD is more active even in the uterus, long before getting any vaccines or sugar. Every child with ADD has a parent with it. ADD is genetic.

Reference.
Wigg K Zai G Schachar R et al. Attention Deficit Hyperactivity Disorder and the Gene for Dopamine Beta-Hydroxylase. *Am J Psychiatry* 2002;159:1046-1048.

* * *

Myth. **Cell phones** cause brain damage or cancer or something.

Fact. No.

Proof. They cause auto accidents for sure, but there has been no sign of brain cancer increasing after cell phones came into use. An interesting recent study published in JAMA showed that holding an active cell phone at the side of the head for 40 minutes caused blood flow in the brain nearest the phone to go up. Much ballyhoo, but (A) that's not brain cancer and (B) last I heard, increasing blood flow to the brain was a good thing.

Reference.
Volkow ND Tomasi D Wang GJ et al. Effects of cell phone radiofrequency signal exposure on brain glucose metabolism. *JAMA* 2011;305:808-813.

Myth. You need eight hours of **sleep**.

Fact. You need what you need.

Proof. In old studies–I can't find them now–studies of how little sleep one needed before performance diminished, there was wide variation between people, and between different ages of people. When I was in graduate school at Harvard, I worked on the scientific subject of sleep. I knew Dr. Dement and other classic sleep experts.

Generally the older you are, the less sleep you need. That's a good thing because very old people don't get much unbroken sleep.

They nap a lot. Teenagers, in contrast, need a lot of sleep. It's wrong to wake them up so early to go to school. Their performance would be enhanced by letting them go to school later.

You reply that the teens *could* go to sleep earlier. True, but just because you go to bed, doesn't mean you can go to sleep. People get sleepy when they get sleepy, whenever that is. It is a bad idea to get in bed for sleep before you get sleepy, because then you are training yourself to be awake in bed.

These are the causes of insomnia in rough order of importance.

1. Psychological stress
2. Lack of physical exercise
3. TV in the bedroom
4. Excessive heat, noise or light in the bedroom
5. Obesity with or without sleep apnea
6. Caffeine, nicotine and other stimulants
7. Rebound alertness from the alcohol drunk at dinner

As I write this America has been jolted by so many pilots and air traffic controllers falling asleep. A tourist bus overturned in Virginia because the driver fell asleep. Insomnia is a big problem nationally. I'm falling asleep writing this chapter. You are falling asleep reading it.

Night jobs are bad, too. After so much evolution, human beings have evolved to be active in the day and to rest at night. The fact that we domesticated fire a long time ago and invented light bulbs has not changed our brain wiring. Many important biochemical cycles are pegged to the light-dark cycle. In fascinating experiments volunteers were kept in furnished underground bunkers for weeks with no way to tell time. Their biological cycles stopped running in parallel; each cycle ran on its own clock. Before long, the cortisol was out of whack with the growth hormone cycle, the body temperature with the catecholamines, etc. Everything out of whack, and the students got fat and sick. Their immune system faltered.

* * *

Myth. Bananas are the best source of potassium

Fact. Bananas are only average for potassium. A raw medium banana has 451 mg. An avocado has 1484 mg, an apple 145, and the other fruits and vegetables spread out in between.

Proof. Many patients given a diuretic by their doctor start to eat a lot of bananas to get extra potassium. Diuretics make people lose potassium in the urine, but eating too many bananas is fattening and constipating. Ripe bananas have the highest glycemic load of any fruit, so they are fattening. And bananas contain kaolin. That's the "kao" in Kaopectate. Bananas are constipating.

Reference. Bowes & Church *Food Values of Portions Commonly Used* 17th edition.

* * *

Myth. People should avoid foods with a **high glycemic index**, like carrots and peas.

Fact. People, authors, nutritionists, doctors, the press, everyone has completely confused the glycemic *index* with the glycemic *load*. Come on, did you really believe carrots and peas were fattening?

Proof. The glycemic *index* is a measure of how rapidly the carbohydrate in a food is absorbed into the blood stream. The glycemic *load* is the product of the glycemic index and the amount of carbohydrate in the food. Peas and carrots have a high index, but a very low load, i.e they contain little total carbohydrate, i.e they are not fattening. In losing weight and monitoring your diet, you should always work with the load, not the index.

Reference. Foster-Powell K Holt SHA Brand-Miller JC. International table of glycemic index and glycemic load values. *Amer J of Clin Nutr* 2002;76:5-56.

* * *

Myth. Aspirin helps prevent stroke, heart attack and death.

Fact. Aspirin may prevent stroke or heart attack a little, very little–it is hard to tell. That's why there have been so many studies. But it definitely increases brain- and stomach-bleeding canceling out any advantage. **Aspirin is only useful in the acute setting of a heart attack-just-starting.**

Proof. None of this is controversial among actual scientists who read literature. Only practicing doctors are confused. But I do mean it–if you have already had one heart attack, keep a small supply of aspirin at the ready to take if you get chest pain again.

References

1. Stavrakis S Stoner JA Azar M et al. Low-dose aspirin for primary prevention of cardiovascular events in patients with diabetes: a meta-analysis. *Am J Med Sci* 2011;341:1-9.
2. Ridker PM, Cook NR, Lee IM et al. A randomized trial of low-dose aspirin in the primary prevention of cardiovascular disease in women. *N Engl J Med* 2005;352:1293-304.

* * *

Myth. Omega-3 fatty acids help prevent heart attacks and strokes.

Fact. A large well-done meta-analysis published in JAMA in August 2012 settled the issue. Omega-3 fatty acid supplements, i.e. fish oil capsules, do not prevent first heart attacks or strokes. That case is closed now, but the book remains open on whether eating fish itself is helpful or whether fish oil capsules can prevent a second heart attack.

Proof. The inspiration for the 1999 Italian study establishing the benefit of omega-3 fatty acids was the long-standing observation that people who eat a lot of fish get fewer heart attacks.[1] That is an epidemiological observation of uncertain provenance. I warned you about those (page 18).

But in this case the scientists did a prospective placebo controlled trial. They gave 1 gram /day of omega-3 fatty acids to patients after a heart attack and followed them for over 3 years.[2,3] They found that, compared to the control, the group getting fish oil saw a reduction in occurrence of death, cardiovascular death, and sudden cardiac death by 20%, 30%, and 45%, respectively. Those are all relative risks, mind you, but it's okay; there is no hint that omega-3 fatty acids cause death on their own, unlike the case with statin drugs. Indeed, omega-3 fatty acids are essential for life.

References.

1. Daviglus ML, Stamler J Orencia AJ et al. Fish consumption and the 30-year risk of fatal myocardial infarction. *N Engl J Med* 1997;336:1046-1053.
2. Marchioli R Barzi F Bomba E et al. Dietary supplementation with *T*-3 polyunsaturated fatty acids and vitamin E after myocardial infarction: results of the GISSI-Prevenzione trial.. *Lancet* 1999;354:447-455.
3. Marchioli R Barzi F Bomba E et al. Early protection against sudden death by T-3 polyunsaturated fatty acids after myocardial infarction: time-course analysis of the results of the GISSI-Prevenzione. *Circulation* 202:105;1897-1903.
4. Simopoulos AP, Robinson J: *The Omega Diet. The Lifesaving Nutritional Program Based on the Diet of the Island of Crete*. New York, HarperCollins, 1999.

5. Rizos EC, Ntzani EE, Bika E et al. Association between omega-3 fatty acid supplementation and risk of major cardiovascular disease events: a systematic review and meta-analysis. JAMA 2012;308:1024-1033.

* * *

Myth. High levels of **homocysteine** in the blood are associated with heart disease.

Fact. It's irrelevant now.

Proof. About the time the association between high levels of homocysteine and heart attacks was revealed, the U.S. government mandated that folic acid be added to bread to prevent neural tube defects in unborn children.[7] An unintended but beneficial consequence of this step was to significantly reduce the national average blood level of homocysteine. Folate in the diet reduces homocysteine in the blood.

Measuring homocysteine in so many people, cardiologists used to put people with high homocysteine on a folate supplement. Now that's not necessary. Remember the Willy family in Myth #11?

After the national blood level of homocysteine declined, however, there was no matching decrease in heart attacks, indicating that while high homocysteine may be associated with heart disease, it is not a cause. Don't confuse association with cause.

Reference. Albert CM Cook NR Gaziano JM et al. Effect of folic acid and B vitamins on risk of cardiovascular events and total mortality among women at high risk for cardiovascular disease: a randomized trial. JAMA 2008;299:2027-36.

* * *

Myth. The **digital rectal exam** in asymptomatic people has reduced deaths from prostate cancer, or morbidity, or something.

Fact. Nope.

Proof. You know the drill by now–institution of the digital rectal exam did not reduce prostate cancer deaths. And finding an enlarged prostate is useless in asymptomatic people. Moreover in a published study, primary care doctors and some urologists were asked to perform a digital rectal exam on a group of men to estimate the size of their prostate. The actual size of the prostate was determined later by ultrasound. There was no association at all between the primary docs' estimates and the actual size! The urologists did better. At least they weren't guessing randomly.

References

1. Roehrborn CG, Girman CJ, Rhodes T et al. Correlation between prostate size estimated by digital rectal examination and measured by transrectal ultrasound. *Urology* 1997;49:548-57.
2. Barclay L Vega C. American College of Preventive Medicine does not recommend prostate cancer screening with digital rectal examination. *Am J Prev Med*. 2008;34:164-170.

* * *

Myth. **America** has the best health care system in the world. Canadians hate their system of socialized medicine. There are long waits for routine surgery. Canadians flock across the border to see American doctors.

Fact. Any American with experience with the American medical system hates it. Indeed, it's the Americans flocking across the Canadian border to buy our own American drugs being sold in Canada for a quarter of the price. Not the Canadians flocking here.

Proof. I shouldn't have to prove my Fact; the people who make statements like the Myth have no proof for their statement. It is only a statement of patriotism. They don't want to debate; they want to fight. I sense their frustration. But anyway, let's do the numbers.

The World Health Organization, part of the U.N., used to produce a listing of the adequacy of health care systems. When that list was last produced in 2000, the U.S. ranked #37, one notch worse than Costa Rica and just beating out Slovenia. Canada came in at #30. France was #1. The WHO ranking was based on life expectancy, child survival up to age 5 years, individuals' experiences with the health care system, and equality of family out-of-pocket expenditures for health care.

The ranking for countries for preventable deaths or "mortality amenable to health care" is more recent, 2008. On that list the U.S. ranked #14. Canada #4, and France #1.

So you don't like the U.N.? How about an American organization? A list prepared by the American National Academy of Sciences in 2004. There the U.S. was #12 on a list of #13, just beating out Germany. We wouldn't beat them now though. Back in 2004, the U.S. ranked #3 for life expectancy; now we are #30.

For this miserable performance Americans pay too much, 17% of their household income or about $7000 per year, far more than any other nation. And that money comes from out-of-pocket or by paying very high insurance premiums. The U.S. is the only developed nation in the world without a single payer system.

The true situation is even worse. The average income per person in the U.S. in 2008 was $45,989. That's what you see in the almanacs, but the figure is misleading because of the grotesque inequality of income distribution in the U.S. The top 20% of Americans have 85% of the income & wealth. The top 10% own 90% of the stock. The vanishing middle class with 15% of the income is pitifully trying to hold on, while the upper class goes on a spending spree.

Mean or average personal income in the U.S. = $45,989
Median personal income = $28,567, about the same as Italy

You get the "mean PI" by dividing all personal income in the country by the total number of earners. You get the "median PI" by knocking out the highest earner and the lowest, repeating the process until a single earner remains; his or her income is the median PI. If everyone makes the same amount, then mean PI = median PI. If the rich get a bigger share, the mean PI exceeds the median PI. That's the case in the U.S.

Did you know, oh American worker, that your income has fallen to match that of the Italians? And you wondered why you felt so poor?

You wondered why you felt so sick? Italians have national health care. Only America lacks a single-payer system of national health care.

The Canadians are not hankering to pay an arm and a leg to see our doctors. They are not flooding across our borders.

References

1. http://www.photius.com/rankings/healthranks.html
2. http://www.allcountries.org/ranks/preventable_deaths_country_ranks_1997-1998_2002-2003_2008.html
3. http://www.worldlifeexpectancy.com/world-rankings-total-deaths

4. http://www.irdes.fr/EcoSante/DownLoad/OECD HealthData_FrequentlyRequestedData.xls
5. Stanfield B. Is US health really the best in the world? *JAMA* 2000;284:483-485.

* * *

And at last, the biggest myth of all . . .

Myth. All disease, and even aging itself, is preventable or curable. From the Declaration of Independence which declares for all men the right to life, liberty and pursuit of happiness, we have inferred a natural right to longevity and feeling healthy.

Fact. Mother Nature was not a signatory to the Declaration of Independence. We are on our own.

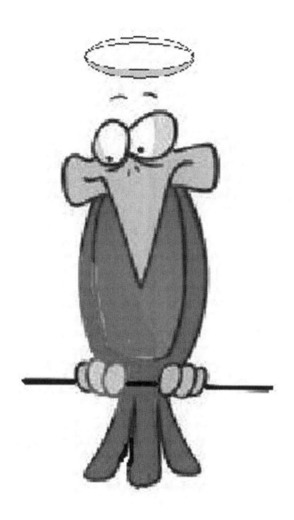

Things Doctors Got Right

FACT #1

....

Antibiotics

Antibiotics were the first really decent medicines doctors ever had.

Why are doctors only half right?

While antibiotics were a huge step in saving mankind from bacterial infections, doctors tend to over-prescribe antibiotics, prescribe them for too long, use expensive antibiotics where a cheaper one would have worked as well, and give antibiotics for diseases that are clearly viral in orgin. This last behavior has contributed to the rise of antibiotic-resistant bacteria, but it's not the worst offender. You will read below what the worst offender is. But first, the wonderful story.

The Story

The first practical antibiotic was sulfonamide. Doctors had long known that bacteria on a glass slide could be stained with dyes to make them more visible through the microscope. They reasoned that if the dyes stuck to the bacteria and to little else, they might be useful in fighting human diseases. The first antibiotic developed this way, a red dye named Prontosil, was synthesized by the Bayer team in Germany (yes, the same Bayer responsible for aspirin) and patented in 1933. The discovery was kept a secret at first by the Nazis.

But then a French scientist discovered that in the body, Prontosil is split into two fragments The antibiotic power belonged to the smaller fragment, sulfonamide. Hence the term *sulfa* drugs, which generations of medical secretaries have misspelled as "sulfur" drugs.

Sulfonamide was already known and widely used in the dye industry. It was off-patent; anyone could make it for free. The German hopes for big profits from Prontosil were dashed impelling them to invade Poland. (Maybe that wasn't the only reason they invaded Poland.)

Sulfonamide saved the life of FDR's son, of Winston Churchill and the life of my father William Anchors. Of the three the most important to me was my father. While stationed in North Dakota during the war, being trained as an Air Force radio operator, my father contracted meningococcal meningitis, the scourge of military bases. At the time it was believed that meningitis was always fatal. The sulfa drugs on the shelf had never been tried on meningitis before. Nothing to lose. The doctors said "Hail Mary" and gave my dad sulfonamide. It saved his life.

Sulfa drugs no longer work on meningococcus; most bacteria have developed resistance to it. The bacteria did not have the chance to do so before, because sulfonamide did not exist in nature until 1903, when human beings synthesized it. I'll talk more about resistance later.

Most people think penicillin was the first antibiotic to be used clinically, but it wasn't, as my father could attest. Penicillin was the second practical antibiotic. The idea for it dated back to 1928 when Englishman Alexander Fleming forgot to put the lid back on a plate of bacteria he was growing. The next day he found the plate contaminated with spots of a blue-green mold. He was going to discard the plate when he noticed a clear circle around the mold where the bacteria had been killed. He grew out the mold and discovered that it was *Penicillium*, the mold that grows on stale bread.

The idea for using penicillin as an antibiotic did not occur to anyone until the Germans publicized their use of sulfa drugs. Fleming knew he had a winner, an English antibiotic, if only he could purify penicillin enough to use it safely in human beings. Mold contain a lot of nasty things besides the good penicillin. That's why you don't eat moldy bread to get over your cold. I hope you don't.

Penicillin was not purified enough for human use until 1940, as a result of a big government research push to develop antibiotics for wounded soldiers. As I said, war was the impetus to develop antibiotics.

Remember, that was back before the large, gluttonously rich pharmaceutical companies as we have now. Before any national government would think of spending tax payer dollars on medical research. The Republicans said, "Why is funding medical research in the national interest? It's the patient's problem and the doctor reaps the reward. Why should the taxpayer foot the bill? Let doctors pay for research."

I'll tell you why. Because developing things like antibiotics requires a group of scientists dedicated to basic research whose daily needs are not paid for by patients. You can't leave the funding of basic research to philanthropic individuals; there aren't enough of them. And you can't reward only positive results. Researchers have to know they will still be paid even if their first scientific idea doesn't pan out. In science, negative results are as important as positive ones. Scientists should not need so much courage to take a risk.

But you can't leave the conduct of research solely up to the pharmaceutical companies either, because their motivation is not the public interest–it's the shareholder's pocket. So governments must get involved in impartially funding basic research. A lesson we learned in 1940 has been forgotten by 2011.

Antibiotic Resistance

Bacteria didn't get where they are today, after four billion years, by being easy pushovers. Among every million bacteria, there are a few mutants with enzymes or other characteristics that might someday, in the right environment, prove useful. Bacteria, you see, have their own tiny Alexander Flemings, and the bacteria wisely fund them. Am I getting too weird?

If the colony is presented with an environmental challenge, such as penicillin in their drinking water, most of the bacteria die. But a few mutant bacteria survive because they happened to have the components needed to resist the penicillin. These mutant bacteria now become the norm, and multiply like crazy. Before long, the whole colony is resistant to penicillin.

This has happened. Most bacteria are resistant to both penicillin and sulfa drugs now. Scientists try to meet the challenge by modifying the original antibiotic to get around the resistance, or developing whole new classes of antibiotics. It's a dynamic business. Sometimes the bacteria get ahead, other times the scientists. It requires a constant infusion of money for research, and vigilance; and we must make sure that talented people go into medical science and stay there. It won't happen if we don't pay them enough. They have families and car payments, too.

Some of our national behaviors tilt the balance against us. One problem is that doctors, lacking medicines for most viruses, give antibiotics to patients who have *viral* disease. Antibiotics don't kill viruses. The doctors are counting on a placebo effect; but that is not moral or legal. To be honest, it's just easier for the doctor to write a prescription for an antibiotic and move on, than to face the anger of the patient being told they will get better on their own. The patient feels stupid then. They had to wait in the waiting room for an hour and anticipate paying the doctor's fee, just to be told they would have gotten better on their own.

The patient still needed to go to the doctor to be sure the disease wasn't bacterial. But American patients, like Americans in general, do not value information or ideas. They want only physical objects, such as bottles of pills. They don't trust ideas. They want only ammo. Gadgets. Things.

You hear a lot about doctors *under*prescribing, or patients not finishing the full course of antibiotic, but that is really NOT a big source of drug-resistant bacteria. Because the antibiotic is still taken in a dose sufficient to wipe out all the bacteria–the normal ones and the mutants, too.

Instead, the two biggest sources of drug-resistant bacteria are:

- Nursing homes, or sick elderly at home without the vigor to eliminate bacteria even with the help of an antibiotic.
- And the really big one! putting antibiotics into animal feed.

In recent decades America has moved its livestock off the farm where the cows ate grass, and chickens ate grubs, to crowded feedlots where the animals are fed nothing but corn, an unnatural diet for them. In this environment the animals tend to get sick. We keep them alive and well, just long enough to be slaughtered for food, by adding antibiotics to their feed. Low levels of these antibiotics are present in your cheeseburgers and chicken tenders. The antibiotics get into your bacteria-filled gut which then becomes a laboratory for developing antibiotic-resistant bacterial mutants.[1]

Notice I'm not giving you many references for all this, because few exist. Who would fund proper studies? Who would publicize the results? Certainly not the government, or farm or pharm companies. They have a financial interest in not knowing. If you read Michael Pollan's excellent book *The Omnivore's Dilemma* and its many sequels, you'll get to the truth.[2]

Most doctors would have added a third item to the above list of sources of drug-resistant bacteria, i.e. treating infections for too short a time. They complain their patients don't take the antibiotics the full ten days prescribed. The patients stop taking the antibiotic as soon as they feel better. But in this case, as in many others, the patients are smarter than the doctor.

Is it really likely–come on–that all the different forms of infection should be treated for exactly ten days? and not say, five or fifteen. What else in Nature is so exact? Really, it's always ten?

Of course not. In fact, in published evidence ordinary urinary tract infections were always cured after the third dose of a sulfa drug. Indeed, the first dose does most of the work. There is no reason to take an antibiotic for ten days for an ordinary bladder infection.[3] There's no evidence that common ear infections benefit from an antibiotic beyond the fifth day either.[4]

For other infections the antibiotic needs to be taken longer. For sinusitis, prostatitis and Lyme disease. In fact, about the only common infection I can think of where ten days is the right duration is ordinary bacterial pneumonia.

The myth that if you don't take the medicine the whole ten days you will relapse is just that, a myth, promulgated by the pharm companies and the doctors to scare you into taking the antibiotics for the full ten days. The pharmaceutical companies do this to make more money. The doctors are just going along.

I should put in my usual disclaimer here. I am NOT your doctor. If your doctor tells you to take an antibiotic for ten says, do it. I'm not going to take the responsibility or be open to anyone's blame.

But between infections, I encourage you and your doctor to read, really read. Honest, the doctors sound like the house sparrows under my roof, chirping, chirping, all the time chirping the same thing. A few hundred years ago, they would have been chirping the Earth is flat, the Earth is flat. But that would not have made the Earth really flat, would it?

- To review . . . Scientific evidence is not the pronouncements of experts. Nothing is true only because someone said so, or because *everyone* said so. Evidence is not the beliefs of an Age.
- It is not the age of a belief either. Precedent plays no role in science.

References

1. Kristof N When food kills. *New York Times* 6/12/2011.
2. *The Omnivore's Dilemma* by Michael Pollan, Penguin Press, New York, 2007.
3. Gleckman RA. Treatment Duration for Urinary Tract Infections in Adults in *Antimicrobial Agents and Chemotherapy* (American Society for Microbiology) 1987, p. 1-5.
4. http://www.mayoclinic.com/health/ear-infections/ DS00303/DSECTION=treatments-and-drugs

FACT #2

Annual Physicals

The yearly physical was a bad idea originally, that turned into a good idea in the hands of a few good primary care doctors who take a lot of time to talk to their patients and teach them.

Why we should have known better

The early universal recommendation to get an annual physical exam did nothing to improve mortality, although it did drive up health costs. The recommendation was promulgated before we had adequate prevention and treatment strategies for most latent diseases. We still don't have them.

How some doctors got un-confused

During the sixties doctors started doing annual routine physicals with chest x-ray, EKG, urine test and increasingly long panels of blood tests. The medical profession made lots of money, but seldom found anything that mattered in *asymptomatic* individuals. For the few things they did find, it would have been just as well to wait until the patient developed symptoms. The outcome of treatment would have been the same.[1]

In the seventies a wave of brilliant college grads entered medical school. They were infected with the philanthropic idealism of the sixties, to be sure, but they were also enticed by the huge profits doctors were making. There's nothing like combining idealism with getting rich to fire up enthusiasm.

But not all of the medical establishment was happy. The health insurance companies and government programs paying the medical bills for the poor and the elderly were very sad ;. They were paying out too much $$. They funded five large studies to see whether routine annual physicals made any difference in morbidity and mortality: the Kaiser Permanent Study, the British, Canadian and Veterans Administration studies. All five studies found that the only things that mattered in the routine physical on *asymptomatic* individuals were:

- blood pressure
- cholesterol
- mammogram
- fecal stool test
- blood sugar
- PAP smear

Readers of this book will know that they were wrong about the first three. Or that there was no adequate evidence for them.

Even I don't know whether picking up low levels of high blood sugar in asymptomatic people makes a difference. I can't find a study for it. People with *very high* blood sugar are not asymptomatic; they didn't qualify to be subjects in the five studies.

The PAP smear was a big success. I will gloat about that later, Fact #5.

On the basis of these five studies, the insurance companies put limits on the routine nonsense, and paid only for the items on the above list.

Then it was the doctors' turn to be ☹. They were making less $$. The best college grads began to pass up medical school and go to business school instead. Some of the business school grads went on to work in the now-hugely-profitable health insurance industry. They were very ☺ there. They made more $$.

Recently some good doctors, seeing the ineffectiveness of routine screening, have taken the radical step of talking to patients for a long time. Some have developed questionnaires, or hired nurses or other personnel to screen patients for symptoms. This idea works because many apparently asymptomatic people are really symptomatic; they just don't recognize that they have symptoms. I wrote a book about this subject, on talking to people, *The Good Doctor.*

The doctors are taught in medical school to use the *history* to come up with the initial diagnostic selection, and then use the *physical* to narrow down the possibilities. Most doctors forget about that. Most doctors don't do an adequate history, so their initial list of diagnoses ranges all over the map. Their physical exam is unfocused. They hope to get the diagnosis from the lab tests or the radiology report, but that way of doing things seldom works.

For the good doctor, there is no substitute for talking to the patient. No substitute for continuing medical self-education and creative thinking. Doctors should have pride in their art. Medicine is a calling, a profession, not a business.

There are some good doctors out there. Go find one for yourself.

References

1. Oken MM Hocking WG Kvale PA et al. Screening by chest radiograph and lung cancer mortality. The Prostate, Lung, Colporectal and Ovarian (PLCO) Randomized Trial. *JAMA* 2011;306:1865-1873. Also read the accompanying editorial on page 1916. Then read other parts of this huge trial showing that screening with current methods is useless except for colonoscopy.
2. *The Good Doctor* by Michael Anchors, Anchors Books, 2010

FACT #3

Colonoscopy

Routine screening with colonoscopy in the U.S. has reduced mortality from colon cancer. [1]

How We Know

By doing screening so frequently, the U.S. is now the only developed nation in the world in which colon cancer mortality has dropped. The mortality has *not* gone down *because* the treatment of established cancer has improved much. (The five year survival may be a little better because of early detection, but the ten year survival is not.) The mortality has dropped because doctors are removing the adenomatous polyps in which colorectal cancer forms.[2]

The story

Many people form little growths, called polyps, in their colon. Most of them are hyperplastic and pose no threat.

But about a third of normal people form a type of polyp called adenomatous polyps. You don't need to know what hyperplastic or adenomatous means. All you need to know is that colon cancer, when it appears, always forms in adenomatous polyps.

About 5% of all American adults develop colon cancer in their life, but that breaks down as follows. The two thirds of people who do not form adenomatous polyps never get colon cancer. The one third that form adenomatous polyps have a 15% chance of getting colon cancer in their life.

About half of the colon cancer victims die from the disease, eventually, though not necessarily within five years. The treatment of colon cancer has hardly improved as noted in Myth #2.

So pending better treatments, the focus has been on preventing colon cancer. The oldest, easiest way to screen for cancers and polyps is the fecal occult blood test which doctors in everyday practice call a "stool guaiac". Guaiac is pronounced *guay'-ack*. Either the doctor or the patient puts some of the patient's stool on a little card and does a chemical guaiac test for tiny amounts of blood the eye cannot see. Cancers and polyps sometimes betray their presence by shedding a little blood into the stool.

Two decades ago, patients with positive stool guaiac were submitted to a barium enema or sigmoidoscopy. If colon cancer was found, the patient went to surgery or chemotherapy, with variable success. If a polyp was found at sigmoidoscopy, it was removed. In this whole process, some people were saved from getting colorectal cancer later by the timely, early removal of an adenomatous polyp.

There were two problems with this program.

- 76% of people with *advanced* colon cancer have negative stool guaiac. The false negative rate is even higher for polyps. In other words, most polyps even in the rectum are missed by the stool guaiac test.

- The sigmoidoscope only reaches one quarter of the colon. Many polyps, and cancers, develop above that point.

As a result of these two problems, old studies with stool guaiacs did not show an improvement in mortality.

Enter the colonoscope. The colonoscope is a long flexible bundle of tiny glass fibers. The operator shines light through some of the fibers and looks through others. The doctor can see the whole colon. Since the procedure is longer in duration than the sigmoidoscopy and the colonoscope must negotiate two 90° turns in the colon, colonoscopy is always done under general anesthesia. There is some risk from the anesthesia, and there are risks of perforation and bleeding. All these risks have been greatly reduced as operators have gained experience, but colonoscopy is still expensive compared to the little guaiac cards. Is it so much better? Yes.

Using the stool guaiacs alone for regular screening and doing colonoscopy only on patients with positive guaiac, you get some reduction in mortality, 15-33% reported. But the analysis in all these studies was flawed because there was no control group. The proper control group would have been to do an equal number of colonoscopies on guaiac negative individuals. The improvement in mortality seen in the guaiac studies may have been due simply to the increased number of colonoscopies done on the guaiac positive people.

The standard of care in this country now is to start routine colonoscopy at age 50 and repeat the study every 5 or 10 years on everyone able to tolerate the procedure. We have dispensed with the stool guaiacs on everybody and started doing colonoscopy on everyone instead. How's that working out?

In a 2009 study from Indiana a group of 715 "average-risk" subjects were given a colonoscopy at baseline.[3] Mean age 61, 59% male, 95% caucasian.[3] Five of the study subjects with colon cancer at baseline were dropped from the study. The remaining 710 were followed for an average of 8 years. Seven *new* colon cancers appeared in the study group. Based on national average data, 21 new cancers would have been expected. There were only 7, so on the face of it, it seems that the colonoscopy reduced the number of cancers by 65%.

The common defect in all such studies is that there is no valid control group. Doctors are so convinced that colonoscopy is good that they are unwilling to do a real control group, that is, a matched group of people designated not to receive colonoscopy at baseline. There are two problems with this approach.

- The Indiana doctors were comparing the frequency of cancers in their 2009 group with a national average calculated *many years before*. What if the baseline rate of cancers had changed?
- No adequate evidence was presented to show that the group of patients chosen for screening were representative of the group in the national survey comparison.

There are no good prospective studies proving that colonoscopy on all-comers reduces colon cancer incidence or mortality. We are left with the fact that (A) we have been doing colonoscopy in the U.S. for god-knows how much money, (B) the treatment of colon cancer itself hasn't gotten much better, (C) but now there are fewer colon cancer deaths in the U.S. and (D) the incidence of colon cancer and deaths is going up in the other developed nations where colonoscopy is not routine.

So I think colonoscopy works. Remember from Chapter 1 the second valid basis for scientific knowledge . . .

- Extensive long-term practical experience accurately observed by many people

Our knowledge about colonoscopy is an example of just this type of empirical knowledge.

I have deliberately *not* talked about whether colonos-copy is cost-effective, because Americans don't under-stand the concept. They are willing to spend any amount of money to save the life of one person, one little dog or one gun. As long as we have all the money we want/need, we make no distinction. Those days are over now, but the truth of our new impoverished situation has not yet sunk into the American consciousness. Maybe my next book can discuss cost-effectiveness. Yes, there is a reason Europeans don't do routine colonoscopy.

What to do now?

Getting a routine screening colonoscopy at age fifty is a good idea, if you can afford it, you can tolerate the procedure and you're not obviously going to die from something other than colon cancer. If *adenomatous* polyps are found and removed, then follow-up colonoscopy is justified.[7]

There is no adequate data to know whether a second colonoscopy is justified if the first one is negative. It depends on the competence and experience of your colonoscopist. If he or she is an old hand, one colonoscopy may be good enough. If he or she is a newbie, you should give the new-bie a second peek in a few years to catch any polyps they missed the first time.

References

1. Stock C Knudsen AB Lansdorp-Vogelaar I et al. Colorectal cancer mortality prevented by use and at-tributable to nonuse of colonoscopy. Gastrointestinal Endoscopy 2011;73(3):435-443.
2. Lakoff J Paszat LF Saskin R et al. Risk of develop-ing proximal versus distal colorectal cancer after a

negative colonoscopy: a population-based study. *Clin Gastroenterol Hepatol* 2008;6:1117-1121.

3. Kahi CJ Imperiale TF Juliar BE et al. Effect of screening colonoscopy on colorectal cancer incidence and mortality. *Clin Gastroenterol Hepatol* 2009;7:770-775.

4. Loeve F van Ballegooijen M Snel P et al. Colorectal cancer risk after colonoscopic polypectomy: a population-based study and literature search. *Eur J Cancer* 2005;41:416-422.

5. Center MM Jemal A Smith R et al. Ward E. International Trends in Colorectal Cancer Incidence Rates. CA 2009;59:366-378.

6. Center MM Jemal A Ward E. International Trends in Colorectal Cancer Incidence Rates Cancer Epidemiology, Biomarkers & Prevention, http://cebp.aacrjournals.org/content/18/6/1688.full.html

7. Lieberman DA, Weiss DG, Veterans Affairs Cooperative Study Group 380. One-time screening for colorectal cancer with combined fecal occult-blood testing and examination of the distal colon. *N Engl J Med.* 2001;345:555-560.

FACT #4

Vaccines

Besides antibiotics, the other great advance in medicine was the development of vaccines.

How We Know

The fact that Americans, today, are so lackadaisical about getting their kids and themselves vaccinated is evidence of the success of the vaccination program. Few Americans alive today have ever seen any of the diseases that doctors prevent so well with vaccinations.

I am 62 years old now. When I was growing up, every child expected to catch chicken pox, measles and mumps at some time. I had all three. Some of the people with those diseases developed pneumonia (chicken pox), encephalitis (measles) and sterility (mumps). In the generation before mine, diphtheria and polio killed and paralyzed many people.

All that is gone now.

But now people have lost their fear of those diseases. They have heard that we stopped vaccinating for smallpox; there have been no natural cases of smallpox in the world since 1978. We are on the cusp of eliminating polio, too. Many Americans wonder why we keep vaccinating children for measles, diphtheria and mumps.

Since the adults have never seen a case of those diseases. They assume that those diseases, too, like smallpox, have disappeared.

Those diseases have not disappeared. As a family practice doctor, I saw some cases of measles and diphtheria. Only the requirement of complete vaccinations to enter school, sixth grade and college has held back the microbiological Mississippi. When England backed off from vaccinating for whooping cough, there were major outbreaks of the disease within two years. England promptly restored the vaccination program.

Unfortunately, the rise of home schooling in the U.S., distrust of government, and the decay of health department funding are all threatening the vaccination system here. If vaccinations are not required, all the gains we've made for children so far will be erased.

That was about kids. American adults, for the most part, don't get flu shots or tetanus boosters. The longer I was in practice, the more my adult patients simply said no. The pneumonia vaccine and shingles vaccine were a hard sell, too.

Let's look at this. What is worthwhile and what is not? I won't look at the childhood vaccines here, because thankfully, they are still required. The pediatric vaccine list keeps changing. You can see the current list at www.cdc.gov. Let's look at the vaccines for adults.

I have already discussed the tetanus shot in Myth #16. Here I will discuss the flu shot, the pneumonia vaccine and the new shingles vaccine.

The Flu Shot

The flu shot aims at preventing influenza, a severe respiratory disease that occurs mainly during the winter months. Flu is a specific disease caused by a specific virus. It is not anytime you have a fever or feel bad. Patients talk about "getting a stomach flu", but that makes no sense. Influenza is a lung disease; what they really had was an intestinal virus. Or they say "I got the flu after the flu shot." What they mean is that they had some chills or a little fever after the flu shot. That's not flu. That's a common mild reaction to the vaccine.

Real influenza is a specific disease with the following symptoms: cough, fever and muscle aches. Other respiratory viruses can cause those symptoms too, but the influenza victims tend to get especially sick, for especially long.

The influenza virus is special among viruses, in that it changes its outer coat each year so that the antibodies formed against it in previous years won't work as well in the new year, or won't work at all. Hence the need to change the vaccine every year.

The influenza vaccine is not totally benign. It is made in eggs; it may contain a little egg protein, so if you are allergic to eggs, don't get the flu shot. Very rarely patients getting the influenza vaccine develop a demyelinating nervous system disease, such as the Guillain-Barré syndrome that developed in 1976 after the CDC came out with a hastily-prepared late-season shot for the swine flu. Swine flu is called "swine flu" because pigs can get the disease, not because pigs cause the disease. Influenza can infect more than one species.

The flu shot is available in two forms, the shot that most people get, and a nasal spray. The nasal spray is more expensive.

In a randomized controlled study, the 1999 flu shot was given to a group of healthy middle-aged volunteers. The control group received a placebo shot of salt water. Neither group of subjects, nor the doctors treating them, knew whether the subjects got the salt water placebo or the real vaccine. Subsequently when the patients were given the flu virus on purpose, 14 out of 31 patients in the placebo group got influenza. In the group that got the standard flu shot only 4 out of 32 got sick, and of those receiving the nasal spray vaccine, 2 out of 29 got sick. The difference between the flu shot and the nasal spray was not significant. Thus the influenza vaccine that year reduced the risk of getting influenza by 76-85%.

Some years the efficacy is worse, some years better. Each year in the spring the CDC has to guess which three epidemic strains of the virus will come through during the next flu season, so that, during the summer, the vaccine industry can produce the needed trivalent vaccine.

In the study above, healthy volunteers were used to avoid the chance of killing anyone. Most deaths from influenza occur in children, immunocompromised people and the elderly. Healthy middle-aged adults are at little risk. For them, it's a matter of convenience; the vaccine reduces suffering and time lost from work. A side-benefit of vaccinating middle-age adults is that it reduces the amount of virus in the population, protecting the kids and elderly. When I was practicing medicine, I noticed that the middle-age adults in families were often eager to get their kids and grandparents vaccinated, but refused to get vaccinated themselves. That makes no sense. It would do the kids and old folks more good for the healthy adults in the house to get vaccinated since the kids and elderly may not get as good protection from the vaccine.

In the future soon, we will have a vaccine against the inside of the virus, the actual DNA, and not the coat. The coat varies from year to year, but the inside stays the same. Once this vaccine is available, we can stop the annual booster shots.

- Treanor JJ Kotloff K Betts RF et al. Evaluation of trivalent, live, cold-adapted (CAIV-T) and inactivated (TIV) influenza vaccines in prevention of virus infection and illness following challenge of adults with wild-type influenza A (H1N1), A (H3N2), and B viruses. *Vaccine* 1999;18:899-906.

The Pneumonia Vaccine, Pneumovax 23

The pneumonia vaccine is mis-named. It is not a vaccine against all forms of pneumonia; it works only against a single form of pneumonia called pneumococcal pneumonia, pronounced *nyu'-mo-kok'-al*, but it's one of the most dangerous forms of pneumonia. In 1900 pneumococcal pneumonia was the most common cause of death in European and American adults. Now, thanks to penicillin, it is seldom fatal, but it still causes deaths among the elderly and immunocompromised people. Muppet master Jim Henson died from pneumococal pneumonia. Deaths among healthy young people are usually the result of a delay in getting to the doctor in time.

Pneumovax vaccine is recommended as a one-time shot for people age 65 or above, or in immunocompromised people of any age. Although pneumococcus is a frequent cause of middle ear infections in childhood, Pneumovax does not prevent ear infections.

- Hutchison BG Oxman AD Shannon HS et al. Clinical effectiveness of pneumococcal vaccine. Meta-analysis. *Can Fam Physician* 1999;45:2381-2393.

The Shingles Vaccine, Zostavax

Shingles is a painful, episodic, blistering skin disease caused by the chicken pox virus. When people get chicken pox as children, they get a few sores on their skin, a few aches and pains, but it's not a big problem. Their body forms antibodies to the chicken pox virus, which stops the disease and ensures that they will never again have *primary* chicken pox with sores all over.

The viral DNA remains, hidden, in the nervous system. Later in life as the amount of antibodies declines, the person can develop *secondary* chicken pox or, as it's called, shingles. In this case the virus reactivates, travels out a single nerve and appears in the skin in the distribution of the nerve. That's why shingles always appears on one side of the body and doesn't extend widely.

Shingles is often associated with burning nerve pain. The older the patients are, the more likely they are to have pain. The pain tends to be worse and may not go away after the skin disease subsides. Pain of this type is called *post-herpetic neuralgia*. To make that word make any sense, I have to tell you that the chicken pox virus and the herpes virus are related.

Zostavax is just a stronger form of the Varivax chickenpox vaccine given to children. It builds up the level of immunity so that shingles does not occur, or if it happens anyway, the disease is much milder. The greatest hope was that the vaccine would eliminate the development of post-herpetic neuralgia, usually the worst consequence of shingles. Unfortunately, while the vaccine is very effective at reducing skin outbreaks, it has not been effective for preventing or stopping neuralgia.

- Chen N, Li Q, Zhang Y et al. Vaccination for preventing postherpetic neuralgia. *Cochrane Database Syst Rev* 2011:16;:CD007795.

FACT #5

PAP Smears

With a wooden paddle like a popsicle stick and a microscope, doctors did the PAP smear regularly and virtually eliminated death from cervical cancer. That's pretty amazing.

How We Know

Greek physician George Papanikolaou developed the PAP smear in 1928. It took twenty years, as usual, for doctors to pick up on its importance, but the test was on hand in time to head off the sharp rise in cervical cancer that resulted from the loosening of sexual mores caused by the Twenties, the Sixties and two world wars. What a horror we would have had, if George had not been so persistent and persuasive. Hats off to him.

Of course his test did have advantages not available to doctors trying to screen for breast and lung cancer. The PAP smear looks at a thin layer of cells on the outside of the cervix. Any doctor can readily access the cervix. Abnormal cells are spotted at a pre-cancerous stage when they can be easily removed, stopping the progression to cancer. Early cervical cancers can be removed before they have time to spread. That was not true of breast cancer, as we saw; and it's not true of lung cancer or melanoma.

The PAP smear is very well tolerated. Painless. Women have been very good about getting their regular PAP smears. If men had to get them, I imagine we'd have seen less compliance.

Worldwide, the recommended age for PAP smears is age 18 to 65. In the U.S. the guidelines say to start Pap smears at age 17 or *whenever the woman becomes sexually active.* The reason the guidelines say this is because almost all cervical cancer is caused by human papilloma virus or HPV, the wart virus. George P didn't know about HPV. You don't have to know about the virus for the PAP smear to work.

146

But the knowledge of the HPV virus allowed us to develop a vaccine. Gardasil works against four types of HPV, two types that cause 75% of cervical cancers and two types that cause 90% of genital warts. The CDC guidelines call for all girls and women between the age of 9 and 26 to be vaccinated. The point is to get the vaccine in, before the girl becomes sexually active.

Question: Dr. Anchors, should a woman who has been vaccinated with Gardasil continue to get PAP smears?

Dr. Anchors: Yes. Because there are other strains of HPV besides the two covered by Gardasil that can cause cervical cancer.

Question: Dr. Anchors, should a woman who has had a hysterectomy, and had the cervix removed, still get PAP smears?

Dr. Anchors. No. Not unless the woman previously had cervical cancer. Some doctors do PAP smears on women post-hysterectomy even if they did not have cancer, but that is wrong. The American Academy of Obstetricians and Gynecologists says so.[1]

Question: At what age can a woman stop getting PAP smears?

Answer: If the woman has had two consecutive negative PAP smears and reached the age of 65, everyone agrees she can stop getting PAP smears.

References

1. http://www.mayoclinic.com/health/pap-smear/AN00013

FACT #6

Smoking Cessation

Steady pressure from doctors got a lot of smokers to quit smoking.

Nothing in recent history has had a greater positive effect on the nation's health. Doctors *can* be leaders. They *can* have an impact. And the tool with which they accomplish so much good is not their stethoscope or their fountain pen; it's their tongue. They have the bully pulpit.

How We Know

If doctors are to get the credit for being leaders in getting people to quit smoking, we must first see if they, indeed, *led*. In the U.S. smoking rates for the general population were 51% in 1950, 43% in 1970, 33.2% in 1980, 25.5% in 1990, 23.3% in 2000 and 21.8% in 2007. The smoking rates for doctors were 51% in 1950 like everyone else, but only 20% in 1975, and 14% 2007.[2] The rates among some medical specialties are even lower. Only 7% of cardiologists smoke, and only 4% of pulmonologists. Clearly, seeing the harm smoking causes had an effect on getting doctors to quit.

So doctors, in their own behavior, were ahead of the curve. Did they and their organizations step forward, early on, to oppose smoking and the tobacco companies? Yes, they did.[3]

Did they have a big impact? Not so much. And here I can't give you a reference because there are no studies of the question. One would have to compare quit rates among a group of patients told by their physician to stop smoking versus a group in which the doctor was mum on the issue. No such study exists from before, and such a study could not be done now since the dangers of smoking are so widely advertised.

My impression is that doctors *did* have a big effect for the good in the 1960-1980 period, however. After that, the public media and the general buzz took over, leading the charge against smoking.

By 2000 we were down to the 20-25% of people smoking, hard core addicts, with the genetic tendency to substance abuse, as we discussed before (page 88). This is a tough group to help. Doctors have come back into the picture, with medications this time, to help the hard-core smokers quit. The hard core addicts "get it" with medicines–it's their thing. Mere talk won't move them. Let's look at the medicines.

Nicotine delivery systems. The gum, the patch, the pipe. These things never made any sense to me. If you were trying to end your addiction to alcohol and I gave you a patch that gave you alcohol, is that going to help? I wouldn't think so, but let's see. Most studies give quit rates like this, from Hays et al.

Success Rates	Placebo	Blind Active	Open Active
At 6 weeks	5.9%	7.2%	10.8%
At 24 weeks	2.8%	5.6%	8.2%

Everyone got a patch. The placebo group, without their knowledge, got the inactive patch. The blind active group got the nicotine patch, but did not know for sure whether their patch was active. The open active group got the active patch and knew it.

So apparently the nicotine delivery systems do help people quit. Hush my mouth. But the most impressive thing overall is how poor the quit rate was, and how transient, without doctor intervention.

There are other tools besides patches–Zyban, Chantix, hypnosis, acupuncture, etc.–but my point is that the most effective tool is the doctor-patient relationship. Look at Wittchen et al. That was a prospective trial in the offices of primary care doctors, 457 patients enrolled. At the end of treatment at 12 weeks the quit rates were 32.8% for advice-only, 35.3% for the nicotine patch and 46.5% for Zyban. At 12-month follow-up, the abstinence rates were: advice-only 29.6%, patch 29.6% and Zyban 29.0%.

The percentage of patients completing the study were: advice-only 56%, nicotine patch 69% and Zyban 79%. Not surprising that more of the nicotine patch patients completed the study, since they were still addicted to nicotine. More of the Zyban patients completed the study, too, because Zyban causes withdrawal effects when stopped. Besides that, these were the heavily-addicted people, who focus on medicines. They come back for prescriptions, but not just to talk.

Even so, the doctor's advice still got 34.8% of the patients to quit in the first place, and that's better than the 10.8% in the Hays trial where the patients were given the patch with no push from the physician. After a year all the gimmicks did no better than the doctor's advice alone.

Doctors should not underestimate their power of persuasion. The good doctor's art is not limited to writing prescriptions.

References

1. www.cdc.gov
2. Garfinkel L Steilman SD. Cigarette smoking among physicians, dentists and nurses. *CA: A Cancer Journal for Clinicians* 2008;36:2-8.
3. Hays JT Croghan IT Schroeder DR et al. Over-the-counter nicotine patch therapy for smoking cessation: Results from randomized, double blind, placebo-controlled, and open label trials. *American Journal of Public Health*, 1999;89:1701-1707.
4. Wittchen HU Hoch E Klotsche J et al. Smoking cessation in primary care - a randomized controlled trial of bupropion, nicotine replacements, CBT and a minimal intervention. *Int J Methods Psychiatr Res* 2011;20:28-39.

Things you learned about statistics in this book

In this book, you learned a lot about statistics as it applies to medicine. Here are some of the terms you learned with the page references.

Apologies

Apologies to Willy, whoever he is, for using his name so often in negative ways.

Sorry for not including more myths about cancer. There must be a lot; I just don't know as much about cancer as I do about cardiovascular disease, obesity and kidney stones.

Sorry for not including more about The Right Diet. I obviously know a lot about the subject. I have published two books, practiced bariatrics for sixteen years and appeared on radio and television. But I'm tired of talking about diet. Nothing would serve the American people better than getting a life, focusing attention on art and people, instead of fixating on their own innards. We are too self-absorbed. There's a world out there! I apologize for saying that.

I apologize to Joel Kauffman for not including his ideas about chelation and fluoridation. I understand that fluoridation of water does no good, but I'm not convinced it does any harm. I included little of Joel's favorable treatment of vitamins and diet supplements. I am on the opposite side of the fence from him on that one. I don't believe Evolution would have left so many average people vitamin-deficient.

I apologize to all the people I offended unintentionally or intentionally in this book. I only wanted the world to be a better place for my three daughters. I wanted the world to contain less foolishness. I wanted life to make sense.

15743509R00088

Made in the USA
Charleston, SC
18 November 2012